THE
fat
RESISTANCE DIET™

REPROGRAM YOUR BODY
TO STAY THIN FOREVER

LEO GALLAND, MD,
AND JONATHAN GALLAND

RODALE

This book is dedicated to

the health and well-being of our readers.

Recipes by Jonathan Galland
Book design by Nicola Ferguson

Library of Congress Cataloging-in-Publication Data

Galland, Leo.
    The fat resistance diet : reprogram your body to stay thin forever / Leo Galland and Jonathan Galland.
        p.   cm.
    Includes bibliographical references and index.
    ISBN-13 978–1–59486–653–1   hardcover
    ISBN-10 1–59486–653–8   hardcover
    1. Reducing diets.   2. Leptin.   3. Inflammation.   4. Obesity—Endocrine aspects.
I. Galland, Jonathan.   II. Title.
RM222.2.G3422 2008
613.2'5—dc22   2007052710

                    2   4   6   8   10   9   7   5   3   1   hardcover

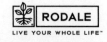

CONTENTS

INTRODUCTION

Welcome to *The Fat Resistance Diet*. You are about to begin an exciting journey to weight loss and a healthy lifestyle—and we have a delicious way of getting you there.

Sweet strawberries
Tart blueberries
Tangy pomegranates

These are just some of the special fat-burning foods that you will enjoy on our diet. Not only will you lose 6 to 10 pounds in the first 2 weeks, you will also be able to say, "I never ate so well in my life!"

This diet shows you how to lose weight by enjoying more satisfying food, with meal plans and recipes that are bursting with freshness and flavor. This is the diet you have been hoping for but never found—until now—because no other diet has our unique combination of cutting-edge science and delicious, all-natural recipes.

We are thrilled to bring you this expanded edition of our book, which we created to fulfill a simple promise: "weight loss without hunger or deprivation." The recipes and meal plans deliver on this promise, giving you a new level of nutrition that reduces inflammation, reverses leptin resistance, and enables weight loss. Our diet has already helped thousands of readers lose weight and discover a healthy new way of life. Readers often share their sense of revelation after following our diet: "Wow! I lost weight and was never hungry."

Our breakthrough concept, that weight gain and the inability to lose weight are caused by a hormonal imbalance called leptin resistance, has captured the attention of the media. Our book has appeared as a cover story in *Fitness* magazine, *Glamour*, *Women's World*, and *First for Women*. Leptin has been recognized as an important part of the weight-loss puzzle in the *New York Times*, the *Wall Street Journal*, and *Time* magazine.

Our diet is having a profound impact on the way many health care professionals view weight loss and healthy maintenance. Physicians on both coasts are recommending our diet to their patients. A major hospital is implementing principles from this book into their patient care and cafeteria. The enthusiastic support of our diet by dedicated professionals is an encouraging sign that advances in nutritional medicine will receive wide recognition by the medical profession in the months and years to come.

This unique diet has been embraced in countries around the world. There are subscribers to our newsletter from Europe, Asia, Africa, and Australia as well as the United States and Canada. Why are they signing up for our newsletter and trying the diet? Because the problems of obesity and diabetes are worldwide, and our book provides a uniquely effective solution.

This book has been translated into the Italian language and published in Italy as *La Dieta Galland*. This is especially gratifying for us as, our family has spent many happy days in the Italian countryside. The fantastic Italian recipes in this book were inspired by the many months we spent living, shopping, and cooking in Tuscany.

The Japanese translation of this book is titled *Dr. Galland's*

Metabolic Diet. This is a particular distinction because very few American diet books are published in Japan. While most diets cannot cross the cultural border, the publisher recognized our cutting-edge science and international recipes and is enthusiastic about bringing our diet to Japan. Jonathan studied Japanese culture and language at a top university in Tokyo. This experience enabled him to use traditional Japanese ingredients such as ginger, green onion, and sesame oil for their amazing health benefits and bold flavors.

But what really motivates us is the same thing now as it has been from the beginning: getting results for our readers—often, spectacular results, such as readers who lost 100, 60, or 23 pounds and lowered their blood pressure or blood sugar.

We understand that adopting a new diet is a challenge, so we made our program as simple, as tasty, and as practical as possible. Our readers often tell us they appreciate how well our diet works for them in the real world. Now, in this special expanded edition, we have added more tools to make the diet even easier and help you overcome every obstacle on your path to success. You'll find more of our favorite recipes, more practical solutions, and more amazing Fat Resistance Foods that supercharge your metabolism. Most of the foods on our diet can be found in your local supermarket, although a few items, such as blueberry concentrate, come from a natural-products store. To make finding these products easier, we created an expanded resource section, which lists producers and retailers. Looking for organic coffee? This section lists organic coffee roasters as well as other natural and organic producers.

Readers love our recipes and have asked for more, so this special edition includes more mouthwatering recipes. These are meals that are fun, flavorful and quick to pull together. That's why it reads like a healthy gourmet cookbook. From the start, Dr. Galland asked his family to help share their passion for delicious and healthy food—and to make it fast, easy, and affordable. Jonathan created over 125 recipes for your enjoyment. Dr.

Galland's wife, Christina, brought her flair and high standards to the wonderful food in this book. Following these special recipes, you can create big, appetite-satisfying flavors using fresh herbs and spices instead of relying on butter or cream.

We grew basil, parsley, sage and chives in flowerpots for the frittatas.
We planted and picked tomatoes for the salsas and gazpacho.
We hit the Union Square Greenmarket for produce fresh from the farm.
We stopped at farm stands to buy local strawberries, blueberries, onions, and arugula.
We chose fresh caught tuna on the docks of a fishing village.
We picked up eggs at the farm.
We searched for exotic spices at the spice market.
We found new and exciting flavors at Asian markets.
We had fun connecting with the people and places that bring us such wonderful, nourishing food.

So go ahead and delight in Green Tea–Crusted Salmon, Blueberry Flax Pancakes, and even Chicken Parmigiano. We understand that by indulging in healthy pleasures, you can stick with this diet and lose weight. That's why the meal plans and recipes reward your efforts to eat healthy by giving you more flavor in each bite.

You'll enjoy fish, chicken, and pasta.
You'll get lots of fresh fruit and vegetables.
You'll have low-fat cheese and yogurt.
You'll delight your palate with new tastes and subtle spices.

And you will take comfort in knowing that this all-natural program is the healthiest diet you can find. No artificial sweeteners or artificial fats are used, because these can interfere with weight loss. No sugar is used, which means sugar cravings will disappear in 2 or 3 days. Instead, our diet gives you high-quality protein, the right fats, fiber, vitamins, minerals, and other key nutrients to support your health. Perhaps you have tried other diets and found them lacking in effectiveness or flavor or difficult to stick with. Don't be discouraged. Our diet takes you to an entirely new place where you can enjoy amazing flavors from around the world while losing weight. So get ready for a sensory journey and discover why our readers are so passionate about our recipes and the results they have achieved. After a few days of eating this way, you will feel refreshed, revitalized, and a little bit lighter.

Please join the growing Fat Resistance Diet community by logging on to www.fatresistancediet.com. Sign up for our newsletter to receive the latest developments about the diet, and start your success story today.

Wishing You Best Health!
Leo Galland and Jonathan Galland

PART ONE

Reversing the Biology of Fat

one

Your Fat Is Not Your Fault

When I first met Lilly, she was thirty-five years old, a respected editor at a national news magazine—and more than fifty pounds overweight. On the medical history form that I give to all my new patients, she had summarized her primary health concern in one brief phrase: "Can't lose weight."

"All my life it's been this way," she told me with tears in her eyes. "Sometimes I can lose for a little while, taking off ten or even twenty pounds. But I have to starve myself to make that happen, and even then, it doesn't last."

Lilly's frustration was all the greater because she'd been following one diet or another ever since high school. In college, she'd supplemented her severely restrictive diet with a vigorous exercise routine. "But even when I dropped a few pounds, I always put them back again—and then some," she explained. "I don't know why I can't lose weight. Even when I'm good, I don't lose much. And if I slip for even a single day, I go up five pounds."

By the time Lilly came to see me, she weighed 214 pounds. Yet as I reviewed her diet and exercise plan, I could see that she was indeed making an effort. Every morning, she worked out for forty minutes—"even on Sundays and holidays," she insisted—and she'd gotten her daily intake down to 1,200 calories or less, mostly in the form of low-fat protein bars, chicken breasts, cottage cheese, and green salads. It was hard to see how she could exercise any more or eat any less. Yet the pounds clung stubbornly to her hips, thighs, and belly.

"Okay, Doctor," she concluded with a sigh. "Tell me what else to cut out. At this point, I'll try anything."

"Frankly," I told her, "I don't want you to eat less. The problem isn't what you're eating—it's what you're *not* eating. So from this day forward, I want you to eat *more*."

Meet the Real Culprit: Leptin Resistance

Like so many other overweight Americans, Lilly was suffering from a condition she'd never heard of—a chemical imbalance that I believe is at the root of our nation's struggle with excess weight. The name of this syndrome is *leptin resistance*—a hormonal dysfunction that disrupts the body's natural ability to regulate appetite and metabolism. Unfortunately, most doctors are not yet aware of this condition. But my decades of clinical practice as an M.D., my success in treating patients with nutritional medicine, and my in-depth exploration of the latest scientific research have convinced me that if you—like Lilly—can't lose your excess weight, then you, too, are probably suffering from leptin resistance.

I believe that the discovery of leptin resistance is the key to freeing millions of overweight Americans from the tyranny of yo-yo dieting, food cravings, and a continual struggle with their weight. Have you ever had the feeling, as you looked at the bathroom scale or tried to button your jeans, that there was something wrong with your body, some stubborn disorder that simply refused to let you shed your excess weight? Well, I'm here to tell you, you were right. If you've tried in vain to lose weight, if you've fallen off every diet you've ever begun, if you've found your healthy intentions sabotaged by sugar cravings and starch binges, you haven't simply been failing or indulging yourself. You're not deficient in willpower or discipline. You're not weak or helpless or out of control. *You're simply suffering from a chemical imbalance*, a chemical imbalance you can correct by cutting out the wrong foods and beginning to eat the right ones.

Our bodies are designed to maintain a healthy weight, without any extra effort on our part. When our bodies are working properly, we eat what we want, and if we inadvertently gain a few pounds, the leptin in our system works to suppress our appetite, increase our metabolism, and reestablish our original weight. This is the mechanism that enables people to stay slim—the natural ability of our bodies to regulate themselves.

The problem comes when this natural ability is disrupted, most often by a condition known as *inflammation*. You may have heard of this syndrome, which has received a lot of attention in the media in recent years. Inflammation contributes to conditions like arthritis, asthma, allergies, and colitis. Many scientists also suspect that it plays a key role in heart disease, atherosclerosis, and cancer. But there's another condition that some scientists now realize is caused by inflammation—obesity. This is because inflammation triggers leptin resistance, which in turn contributes to a sluggish metabolism, unchecked cravings, and, eventually, unwanted pounds.

Inflammation is part of your body's response to many different types of stress, including infection and injury. Sometimes inflammation creates visible signs and symptoms: redness, swelling, heat, and pain. Sometimes it's visible only on a cellular level, so that you—and your doctor—may not even be aware that you have it. But it's present more often than you might suspect; in fact, recent research has found two new causes of inflammation—the type of food you eat and excess weight itself.

So, I told Lilly, your body can get caught in a vicious circle. Inflammation disrupts your body's natural weight regulation system. As a result, you gain weight. Then the excess fat creates more inflammation, making the extra weight unusually difficult to lose. That's why, once begun, weight gain often continues. The weight itself is worsening the condition that caused you to put on weight in the first place.

If you've been a lifelong dieter, you've probably noticed this pattern yourself, without realizing what was causing it. Most people don't stabilize at a single unhealthy weight. Unless, like Lilly, they diet and exercise strenuously, they find that their weight has a tendency to increase. Sometimes they succeed in losing a few pounds—but they usually gain back more than they lost.

I'll explain leptin resistance and the link between inflammation and weight gain more fully in Chapter 2. For now, understand this: your weight problem is not a matter of will or discipline, but a chemical imbalance that, once corrected, holds the key to permanent weight loss. The good news is that this imbalance can be fairly easy to correct, simply by changing the foods you eat.

Once you make this change—adding the right fruits and vegetables, nuts and seeds, and protein sources, and cutting back on sugar and unhealthy fats—you'll notice a remarkable change. Not only will you feel better and look better and find the pounds dropping almost effortlessly, but you'll also stop craving unhealthy foods. Most diets are based on what you can't have. In contrast the Fat Resistance Diet is based on a philosophy of fulfillment, providing your palate with all the tasty, delicious, and satisfying food you could ever want. True, burgers and fries are not on the Fat Resistance Diet, but once your taste buds are reawakened and your body reenergized, "fulfillment" takes on a new meaning. You won't feel hungry, and you won't even feel as if you're on a diet. I know, because I myself eat this way, and it's very satisfying. I'm able to say those magic words that everyone wishes were true: I eat whatever I want, and I never gain weight. If you follow the Fat Resistance Diet, within a few weeks, you'll be saying them, too.

Restoring Your Body's Natural Balance

Lilly was skeptical. But she agreed to give the Fat Resistance Diet a try. I explained to her the basic principles behind the diet: inflammation can be set off by eating certain foods, which she needed to avoid. But inflammation can also be cured by eating other types of foods, so she actually needed to eat more of those. Unfortunately, most American diets are rich in inflammatory ingredients and sadly lacking in anti-inflammatory nutrients. Red meat, white flour, sugar, and hydrogenated fats all inflame your body; so do French fries. On the other hand, berries and cherries, walnuts and almonds, whole grains, and fish help to heal inflammation, as do cabbage, broccoli, garlic, and flaxseeds. In the following chart, you'll find a list of the Top 40 Superfoods that will fast-track your cure for inflammation and enable you to lose weight.

When Lilly heard that I actually wanted her to eat *more,* she couldn't believe it. "You don't lose weight by eating more," she kept insisting. But I assured her that the Fat Resistance Diet was based strictly on mainstream science: cutting-edge research conducted by scientists at Harvard, Johns Hopkins, and Rockefeller universities, published in respected medical journals such as *JAMA,* the *Journal of the American Medical Association.* I'd prescribed versions of this diet to hundreds of patients, each of whom had gone on to lose substantial amounts of weight. Following my diet, they had achieved their ideal weight and avoided regaining the weight they'd lost.

Lilly agreed to follow an early version of the Fat Resistance

Top 50 Fat Resistance Foods

These foods will help fast-track your weight loss by healing your inflammation and restoring your sensitivity to leptin. They are used abundantly in all three stages of the Fat Resistance Diet, so if you follow the meal plans and recipes, you'll be getting plenty of fat resistance foods.

BEVERAGES (UNSWEETENED)

Blueberry juice

Cherry juice

Green tea

Pomegranate juice

Vegetable juice

NUTS AND SEEDS (FRESH, UNSALTED, NOT ROASTED)

Almonds

Flaxseeds

Sesame seeds

Walnuts

FRUIT (FRESH)

Apples

Blueberries

Cherries

Grapefruit

Kiwi

Oranges

Peaches

Pomegranates

Red grapes
   (organic)

VEGETABLES

Arugula

Asparagus

Bell peppers

Bok choy

Broccoli

Cabbage

Carrots

Kale

Leeks

Onions

Romaine
   lettuce

Scallions

Shiitake
   mushrooms

Spinach

Swiss chard

Tomatoes

SEA VEGETABLES

Kombu

Nori

Wakame

HERBS AND SPICES

Basil

Black pepper

Cardamom

Chives

Cilantro

Cinnamon

Cloves

Garlic

Ginger

Parsley

Turmeric

FISH

Flounder

Salmon

Sole

Tilapia

OTHER

Egg whites

Yogurt (plain,
   nonfat)

Diet. To her joy, she soon began to lose weight at the rate of five pounds a month. (If you follow the plan laid out in this book, you can lose weight even more quickly—ten pounds in the first month, and five to ten pounds a month thereafter.)

Half a year later and thirty pounds lighter, Lilly was able to fit into her favorite jeans. But she didn't stop there. Sticking to the Fat Resistance Diet enabled Lilly to lose an additional four or five pounds a month, even though she was eating more food—and more types of food—than she had throughout her years of dieting.

By the time she'd been on the Fat Resistance Diet for one year, Lilly's weight had dropped to 150 pounds—the lightest she'd been since the age of fifteen. "I feel better than I've ever felt," she said in amazement. "Everyone tells me I look terrific— and not just because of the weight. My skin, my hair, even my fingernails all feel healthier. I'm calmer, I have more stamina, and I'm sleeping better than I have in years."

Yes, I told her, those were all the effects of curing her inflammation. Obesity is only one result of a condition with many side effects, including skin problems, thinning or lackluster hair, indigestion, gas, bloating, sleep problems, irritability, and depression. Curing the underlying inflammation had not only healed Lilly's weight problem but also had resolved her other symptoms as well— symptoms she hadn't even realized were linked to her obesity.

Best of all, she concluded, was her newfound trust in herself and her eating choices. "Before, I felt I was always on the verge of losing control," she told me. "Now, I can indulge my love of food and enjoy eating. I'm at peace with what I eat and at peace with my body. I never thought I could feel this way—and I feel this way all the time."

Discovering the Fat Resistance Diet

By now, you may be ready to turn to Part Three and start following the Fat Resistance Diet—and if that's how you feel, go right ahead. The three stages of this eating plan have been carefully designed so that you can simply follow the recipes and meal suggestions without having to think further about what you eat.

But if you, like Lilly, want to know more, read on. I will tell you how I discovered the Fat Resistance Diet, and why I am so certain that it will bring you a lifelong healthy weight.

The story begins almost twenty-five years ago, soon after I started practicing as an internist. I had always been a problem solver—someone who enjoyed looking at a situation and figuring out how to make it better. So when patients began coming to me with problems that other doctors hadn't been able to resolve, I started looking for new solutions.

As I explained in my first book, *Superimmunity for Kids*, I soon realized that many of the problems I was seeing—from arthritis to asthma—were related to a faulty immune system, which had in turn been impaired by a deficiency of essential fats in the American diet. Most doctors at the time had no knowledge of essential fats, largely because the groundbreaking research on fish oils had not been popularized.

Fortunately, I was aware of these new scientific breakthroughs for two simple reasons: I had an interest in nutrition, and I kept up with the scientific literature. I'd had a very challenging professor in medical school—one who had insisted that we learn not only how to treat patients but also how to interpret the science that had produced new treatments. In fact, he taught us, the generally accepted interpretations of cutting-edge research are often incorrect. Many medical protocols are too simplistic or represent a misunderstanding of what the research means. If we were to be effective physicians, we would have to keep up with the research ourselves. Only then could we be sure that our patients were benefiting from the most current scientific knowledge.

I put his teachings to good use as I began to review the latest scientific research on the biochemistry of inflammation and its relationship to a wide variety of immune disorders, including asthma, allergies, arthritis, joint pain, fatigue, and colitis. I soon realized that a lack of omega-3 oils and other essential fatty acids was at the root of many of my patients' problems, and that their conditions could be healed with proper nutrition.

In the course of prescribing the seeds, nuts, fish, and oils that contained the healing fats my patients needed, I began to notice something interesting. Not only would my patients show improvement in their "presenting condition"—the asthma, arthritis, or colitis that they had come to me to heal—but they would also feel better generally, more energetic, relaxed, and clear-headed. Many of them told me they no longer struggled with depression, that they had resolved long-standing sleep problems, or that they were getting compliments on their hair and skin. And many of them, without even trying, had begun to lose weight.

Of course, many of my patients *were* trying to lose weight. Throughout the 1980s and early 1990s, I had numerous patients who were following Pritikin and similar low-fat diets that were popular at the time. The ten years that followed were marked by Dr. Robert Atkins and the low-carb eating plan. As time went on, I began to notice that both approaches, while not particularly successful at long-term weight loss, were leaving my patients with a disturbing set of side effects: fatigue, constipation, bloating, gassiness, skin problems, menstrual problems, joint pains, dry hair, brittle nails, irritability, sleep problems, and depression. It became clear that these symptoms were the result of nutritional deficiencies. While the low-fat diets tended to be deficient in essential fats, low-carb dieters were lacking in the fiber and plant-based nutrients that their immune systems needed to function. As a result, their bodies were struggling to overcome inflammation and its related symptoms—but they didn't have the nutrients they needed to accomplish this essential task.

To make matters worse, my patients were unable to lose weight permanently with these other diets. Even when they were following the diets, they reported constant cravings for starches, sweets, or other forbidden foods. And as soon as they ended the most restrictive portion of the diets—particularly on low-carb regimens—they found themselves not only regaining their lost weight but often adding a few more pounds as well.

So I began working with these patients on two levels. First, I would address their inflammation, which I had come to see as the root cause of both their illness and their obesity. Second, I would help them lose weight, because new research was indicating that excess weight itself was a primary cause of inflammation. If we didn't heal my patients' inflammation, they would continue to be obese. And if they remained obese, their excess fat would set off a new round of inflammation. Clearly, these two problems had to be solved together. The solution I devised was the Fat Resistance Diet.

The Fat Resistance Diet: An Individualized Plan

My first step was to give each patient an individualized questionnaire with detailed inquiries regarding his or her food habits. Utilizing research done at the National Institutes of Health, I developed computer software that would make it easy for people to analyze the nutritional quality of their own diets. That software, called the Nutrition Workshop, is now being used at the Johns Hopkins School of Medicine to train medical students—and you can find it at www.nutritionworkshop.com. Together, my patients and I used the software to analyze the dietary choices that were getting them into trouble and to discover the nutritional solutions that would help them heal.

What this process taught me was something I had suspected all along: there is no single dietary program that's right for everyone, especially when it comes to the need for carbohydrate or protein. Most of the popular diets of the last two decades have mandated a strict protein to carbohydrate ratio, either high protein or high carbohydrate. But I have many patients who need high-protein diets to feel their best. If they don't get 35 percent of their daily calories in the form of protein, they'll feel light-headed, irritable, and fatigued. Others feel sick if they try to process that much protein in a single day, experiencing lethargy, depression, and digestive problems. These special nutritional needs are not just the result of adjusting to a change in diet; they are enduring characteristics of each person. Nutritional scientists have become increasingly aware of the varying dietary protein needs of different people, which is why the National Academy of Sciences has recommended a remarkably broad range of protein consumption—from 10 percent to 35 percent of our daily calories.[1] In developing the Fat Resistance Diet, I've incorporated these differences in the design of the diet's three stages, with Stage 1 having the greatest amount of protein and the highest protein to carbohydrate ratio, for reasons explained in Chapter 6.

I also learned that there are some foods that inflame our bodies fairly consistently, while other foods are generally effective at healing the inflammation. And excess body fat itself is a source of inflammation, as well as a product of it. So if the Fat Resistance Diet was to provide a long-term solution to obesity, it needed to steer us toward healing foods and away from those that might make inflammation worse.

With these guidelines in mind, I gradually developed an approach to eating that could work for all my patients, all of the time. The Fat Resistance Diet gives us a lot of flexibility in choosing the foods we need. But it also helps us make healthy choices that avoid foods that will guarantee weight gain.

Escaping the Toxic Food Environment

The concept of the "toxic food environment" has been proposed by Dr. Kelly Brownell, a psychologist at Yale University who works with severely obese patients.[2] Dr. Brownell points out that the American diet is shaped by the extraordinary availability of high-calorie, low-nutrient food, much of which has been carefully engineered to stimulate and then satisfy cravings. As a result, the American palate has been conditioned to a high-fat, high-sugar, and high-starch diet, an approach to food that can quickly become addictive.

Think of a teenage boy who likes to turn the stereo up full blast. Pretty soon, he can't be satisfied by softer music. If the loud music isn't blasting, he doesn't feel satisfied. He almost literally loses the capacity to appreciate softer, more subtle sounds, needing an ever-louder, more insistent noise to satisfy his musical tastes.

As far as food is concerned, we've become a bit like that teenage boy. Just as he needs a loud blast of music, we need the quick fixes of fat, starch, and sugar that flood our taste buds, fill up our stomachs, and cause our hormones to spike in quick rushes. Then, when those sugar highs lead to punishing crashes, we feel a ravenous hunger that only another high-fat, high-sugar meal will satisfy.

But suppose we take that teenager and put him in the middle of a country field. At first, he might miss the pounding bass and deafening drums to which he's grown accustomed. But after a while, his ears might become attuned to the quieter sounds of birds singing and wind rustling through the tall grass. He might come to enjoy the rhythms of the cicadas and the creaking of the tree frogs. The country sounds, at first almost imperceptible, might come to seem quite loud, varied, and, ultimately, fascinating.

That's the experience people have on my diet, only instead of their ears becoming more sensitive, it's their taste buds that open up to delightful new flavors. Where once you could be satisfied only by the crude sweetness of refined sugar or artificial sweeteners; now you can savor the tart subtleties of fresh blueberries or the crunchy texture of green apples, while such herbs as rosemary, basil, and fresh parsley become exquisitely intense. "It's as though I can taste the colors," one of my patients told me, describing her experience of eating the Mexican Salad in Stage 1 of this diet. "I never thought a diet would make me enjoy food *more.*"

As I watched my patients adapt to the Fat Resistance Diet, I realized that most of us need a transition from the toxic food environment to a healthier set of surroundings. We need to reprogram our body chemistry from its unhealthy condition of inflammation to the state designed by nature, in which our appetite, metabolism, and food choices all work together to effortlessly maintain a healthy weight. Ultimately, our goal is to tap into our body's inner wisdom about what kinds of nourishment we need. But that wisdom may need a little time to make itself heard over the noisy claims of trans fats, sugar, and refined starch.

The Fat Resistance Diet: A Three-Stage Program

To help you make the transition—and to provide the reinforcement of a quick initial weight loss—I created three stages for the

---

JONATHAN'S KITCHEN TIPS:

FRUIT ON THE COUNTER

We're excited to start off with a tip that can help you escape the toxic food environment. It's a simple and effective way to eat more fruit. Place a bowl or basket on your kitchen counter, and fill it with seasonal fresh fruit such as oranges, apples, blueberries, or cherries. Every time you walk into the kitchen, you'll have a reminder to enjoy a piece of fruit. During citrus season, I like to keep a bowl of oranges, clementines, or tangerines on the counter, along with a bowl of bright green limes. Everyone grabs them for snacks or dessert, which means we eat more fruit. Seeing the limes encourages me to wake up salads and other dishes with a squeeze of fresh lime juice. Enjoy!

Fat Resistance Diet. Each stage is designed to help you overcome leptin resistance, heal your inflammation, and reprogram your body to automatically regulate your weight—its natural state.

Stage 1 jump-starts the process of healing inflammation and overcoming leptin resistance. It's also designed to lower insulin levels and reduce insulin resistance. I'll explain the connection to insulin resistance more fully in Chapter 5, but for now, just remember that eating a diet high in sugar and refined flour, besides contributing to the process that creates leptin resistance, has also left many of us with uncontrollable food cravings that are hard to resist. These cravings are not the body's natural wisdom but are more like an addiction that must be broken. The food choices in Stage 1 are designed to do just that, while enabling you to lose six to ten pounds in the first two weeks.

Some of my patients enjoy Stage 1 so much, they don't feel the need for any other diet. If you're like them, feel free to remain on Stage 1 for the rest of your life. It has all the nutrients you need to stay healthy. But if you'd like to add more food choices to your diet after your initial "reprogramming," move on to Stage 2.

Stage 2 is the long-term weight-loss part of the Fat Resistance Diet. Now that the first stage has righted your chemical balance and begun to address your leptin resistance, Stage 2 gives you a chance to eat a wide variety of delicious foods that will leave you feeling satisfied—and slim. You'll lose about two pounds a week on Stage 2, and you can remain at this stage as long as you like: its healthy food choices will continue to heal your inflammation and help your body use leptin more efficiently. (You can read more about how this works in Chapter 2.) I recommend remaining at Stage 2 until you're at or close to your healthiest weight. Like Stage 1, this stage is designed to be a satisfying, sensual experience, offering you chef-quality recipes and a wide range of flavors.

Stage 3 is your lifelong weight maintenance program, an eating plan that will protect you from inflammation and keep your leptin resistance at bay while encouraging you to sample a delightful array of tasty foods. Frankly, if you're willing to lose weight more slowly, you can go right to Stage 3, knowing that eventually your inflammation will heal, your leptin resistance will abate, and your healthy weight will restore itself. Most people, however, want to lose weight more quickly, so I recommend undertaking this diet the way it was designed.

All three stages of the plan are designed to leave you feeling satisfied and full, training your palate and your taste buds to derive more pleasure from every bite. Have you ever kept eating after you felt full, simply because you hadn't yet satisfied your desire for something delicious? You won't have that experience on the Fat Resistance Diet! Instead, like Lilly, you may feel that you are eating more "richly" and feeling more satisfied than you ever have before.

In fact, as I've watched hundreds of patients do well on this eating plan, I've been struck by how eagerly they welcome this new approach to food. "Why would I go back to eating the way I did before?" one patient asked me. "It would be like returning to a neighborhood where there were toxic fumes. When you live in a place like that, you tend not to notice the smell—but when you've been away and return, it starts to make you sick. I could no more eat the way I used to than I could voluntarily go stand behind a bus and breathe in the exhaust."

Why Other Doctors Don't Tell You About Leptin Resistance

After only a month on the Fat Resistance Diet, Lilly couldn't believe her results. Not only had she lost weight, but her whole body felt slimmer and tighter. She'd already begun to enjoy a boost of energy and to appreciate her glowing skin and revitalized hair.

"Why are you the first person to tell me about this diet?" she demanded one day. "If it's so healthy, then why doesn't every doctor know about it?"

I explained to Lilly what I've already explained to you: the Fat Resistance Diet is supported by groundbreaking studies conducted at Harvard and Rockefeller universities, where biologists, chemists, and geneticists have been unraveling the secrets of human hormones. Their discoveries—which I explain more fully in Chapter 2—have profound implications for weight loss and health. Research on leptin resistance is so fresh and new that most doctors are not even aware of its existence. Someday, I believe, every physician will know about them—or at least will know about the treatment protocols that they imply. As a result, the Fat Resistance Diet is the only eating plan based on the latest scientific knowledge about how our bodies gain and lose weight.

Becoming Your Own Diet Doctor

When I had been in practice for about five years, a remarkable thing happened. One of my patients, whom I hadn't seen for at least two years, returned for a routine checkup. Naturally, I asked him how he'd been, and he told me that the previous winter, he'd started to get sick.

"I thought about calling you," he explained. "But then I realized that I already knew what you'd suggest. So I went ahead and took care of myself."

Perhaps if this man had been the only patient to tell me such a story, I wouldn't have thought much of it. But over the years, more and more patients have returned with similar accounts. They'd come to me and found a cure—in some cases after years of illness. Then they went home and took care of themselves.

I suppose if enough of my patients learn this lesson, I'll become obsolete! But it's an obsolescence I'll welcome, because nothing is more satisfying to a physician than to know that his patients are able to heal themselves.

So I've designed this book to give you two choices. One is simple—turn to Part Three, follow the meal plans and recipes, and allow your body to regain its natural weight-loss ability. Even if you never understand why or how this diet works, you'll soon find yourself intuitively choosing healthy foods and avoiding items that will make you sick. Without necessarily being able to explain your choices, you'll have become your own diet doctor.

But if you want to learn more, this book will help you understand every feature of the Fat Resistance Diet. In Chapter 2, you'll get a short course in inflammation, leptin resistance, and a newly discovered hormone called adiponectin. When you've finished reading, you'll be able to visualize just what's going on in your body when you gain, lose, or maintain your weight. You'll understand exactly why you're making the dietary choices I recommend in Part Three—always a powerful factor in sticking with a new diet.

Then you'll master the principles of the Fat Resistance Diet. Chapter 3 will explain what kinds of fats can interfere with weight loss—and which types can actually help you lose weight. Chapter 4 will dispel the myths about carbs, helping you see why some high-carbohydrate foods can be among the most slimming food choices you can make. And in Chapter 5, I'll contrast my approach with today's popular diets. This chapter will make it clear why only the Fat Resistance Diet offers a permanent—and satisfying—solution to weight loss.

Part Two outlines the practical weight-loss advice of the Fat Resistance Diet. In Chapter 6, you can read about the three stages of the Fat Resistance Diet: Stage 1—an initial rapid weight loss of six to ten pounds in two weeks; Stage 2—achieving your ideal weight through a loss of two pounds per week; Stage 3—maintaining your ideal weight for the rest of your life. Following the Fat Resistance Diet will reawaken your joy in food, freeing you from the tyranny of calorie-counting and unsatisfied cravings. Not only will you achieve and maintain your ideal weight, you'll take enormous pleasure in doing so.

Also in Part Two, I explore some other sources of inflammation and some additional tools for healing. Chapter 7 shows how a lack of physical activity promotes inflammation, and sets out some easy-to-follow recommendations for strengthening and toning your body. Just as the Fat Resistance Diet helps you to enjoy food again, this approach to exercise is designed to help you recover the joy of movement.

Chapter 8 will help you understand how stress is another source of inflammation, and thus another factor in your weight gain, while also offering some powerful de-stressing exercises. Chapter 9 demonstrates how toxins inflame your body, and explains why the Fat Resistance Diet is the first step in detoxification. And in Part Three, you'll find the meal plans and recipes that allow you to put the Fat Resistance Diet into practice.

I firmly believe that the body knows what it needs—although sometimes, particularly in our modern world, it can lose touch with its own innate wisdom. My goal is to help your body regain its natural knowledge, and that is precisely what the Fat Resistance Diet is designed to do. After you've eaten this way for a few weeks, you will know what to eat in order to lose weight. All you'll need to do is follow my eating plan and listen to your body—which will repay you with your shedding pounds effortlessly, even as it offers you more pleasure from food than you've ever had.

Summary of Chapter One:
Your Fat is Not Your Fault

1. If you are struggling with your weight, it is not your fault.

USING FRESH HERBS

Our readers have told us what is important to them: delicious, easy-to-prepare food and getting weight-loss and health results. That's why our recipes are brimming with fresh herbs such as parsley, basil, and cilantro. Chefs throughout the world bring amazing flavor to dishes simply by showering them with these herbs. But these little herbs also pack a big nutritional punch that can help knock out inflammation. Here's how to get started with herbs: Pick up a bunch of fresh parsley, basil, or cilantro in the vegetable aisle at the supermarket. Look for bright green leaves, and skip anything wilted. When you are making something in the kitchen, pull off a handful of fresh herbs. Rinse them well and pat dry, then give them a chop. Sprinkle on dishes such as omelets, salads, chicken, fish, and sandwiches. Once you get started, using chopped herbs becomes an easy and enjoyable part of your daily routine.

2. Weight gain and the inability to lose weight are caused by a hormonal imbalance called leptin resistance.
3. The key to permanent weight loss is reversing leptin resistance by eating plenty of Fat Resistance Foods.
4. The Fat Resistance Diet helps you escape the toxic food environment and enjoy a healthy new lifestyle.

two

Leptin Resistance: The Reason You Can't Lose Weight

Kate was a forty-five-year-old single mom who came to see me because she was constantly getting sick. She had two kids, ages eight and ten, and she seemed to catch any infection they brought home—colds, sore throats, and flu. But while her children bounced back quickly, Kate struggled with each illness, and her weight fluctuated with her health. Over fifteen years, Kate had gradually put on forty-five pounds, and when she came to see me she weighed 180.

Despite Kate's frustrations with her weight, that wasn't why she'd come to see me. Her main concern was the latest respiratory infection, which included a cough, fatigue, and shortness of breath whenever she exercised. She had started taking medication for bronchitis, but it didn't seem to be helping.

When I asked her about her weight history, Kate explained that she'd always been very active as a teenager, when she had loved to play tennis and hike. The exercise, she thought, had been successful in keeping her weight down, as had her sense of portion control. "I tell my kids the same thing," she explained. "Eat whatever you want in moderation, just don't stuff yourself."

And indeed, when I analyzed Kate's diet, I saw that she averaged about 1,700 calories a day, which seemed like a reasonable intake for a woman of her size. Nevertheless, her weight had continued to increase.

"I'm confused," Kate said finally. "Why are you asking me so much about my weight? I know I need to lose a few pounds, but that's not why I'm here."

On the contrary, I told her. The same condition that was producing her series of illnesses was causing her to gain weight. And the same diet that would build up her immune system would also solve her weight problem.

I pointed out that in order to keep her caloric intake down, Kate had been skimping on fruits and vegetables in order to leave room for "a few low-sugar cookies," "a little low-fat ice cream," and other nutritionally poor "diet foods." Her deficiency in plant fiber and omega-3 essential fatty acids was wreaking havoc with her immune system, which was why she kept getting sick. But her dietary shortcomings were also disrupting her body's delicate biochemical balance and sabotaging her metabolism. As a result, she was slowly but steadily gaining weight.

"So what I'm eating is making me sick—and making me gain weight?" Kate asked.

"Something like that," I replied. "Though frankly, I'm more concerned with what you're *not* eating. I believe you're suffering from a condition known as inflammation, a bodywide disorder that impairs the immune system and can be cured through nutritional medicine—that is, by adding the right foods to your diet."

"Inflammation?" Kate asked, bewildered. "But I don't have any redness or swelling or fever—at least, not when I'm not sick."

That was correct, I told her. The inflammation from which she suffered operated on a cellular level and often had no obvious symptoms. Her susceptibility to illness and her slow but steady weight gain, however, were telltale signs that her immune system had been compromised by inflammation. And her body would not be able to heal this underlying disorder without the essential nutrients that were missing from her diet.

I told Kate about a study done in Italy in which children with recurrent respiratory infections had been given a small dose of flaxseed oil for several months. Flaxseed oil is rich in omega-3 essential fatty acids as well as in carotene, the plant-derived form of vitamin A. Compared to a control group of children given placebo capsules, the flaxseed group had fewer, milder, and shorter infections.[1] I told Kate that if she followed the diet I gave her—rich in omega-3 fats as well as in vitamins—she might expect the same results.

"But how does this affect my weight?" Kate wanted to know.

I explained that besides disrupting the immune system, chronic inflammation sets in motion a chain of biochemical events that results in a hormonal imbalance called *leptin resistance*, a condition that makes it nearly impossible to maintain a healthy weight. "So when we cure your inflammation," I concluded, "your leptin resistance should also disappear. Both your weight issues and your respiratory problems should resolve."

It took a while for Kate to see the connection between getting sick and gaining weight—a link that no other doctor had ever mentioned to her. But she was willing to begin a diet plan that I developed for her, including ground flaxseeds, walnuts, and lots of fruits and vegetables. Now, instead of dietetic cookies and ice cream for dessert, Kate was enjoying Fruit Kebabs with Pomegranate Glaze, Baked Apple with Cinnamon and Walnuts, and Strawberry Mango Granita. At least twice a week, she had a bowl of my Immune Power Soup with carrots, leeks, onions, garlic, parsley, fresh basil, shiitake mushrooms, and chives. I gave her recipes for incorporating smoked salmon (rich in omega-3 fats) and a wide variety of vegetables into healthy omelets and frittatas.

To her amazement, Kate made it through the next two months of winter without picking up any new infections, and she went through the following winter with only one short-lived cold. But she was even more surprised to realize that, without any additional effort on her part, her weight had started to drop. True, she was now able to exercise more. But even more significant was the way her new diet had addressed the underlying condition that had been sabotaging her other weight-loss efforts. By the time I saw Kate for a checkup the following winter, she had lost the forty-five pounds she had gained since turning thirty.

We were also able to measure the improvement in Kate's chronic inflammation using a blood test for CRP, or *C-reactive protein*, a protein produced in the body in response to certain kinds of inflammation. CRP has received a lot of attention in the press because of the many studies showing a link between elevated levels of CRP and the development of heart disease, high blood pressure, and diabetes. When I first saw Kate, her CRP was elevated at 7.52 milligrams/liter, indicating a significant amount of inflammation. After a year without illness and a weight loss of forty-five pounds, Kate's CRP measured less than 1 milligram/liter, an excellent reading that revealed our success in not only boosting her immunity and helping her to lose weight, but also curing the underlying condition at the root of both problems.

"I wasn't really trying to lose weight," she kept repeating. "And the whole time I followed your plan, I was never even hungry! Your diet is amazing!"

Kate's story is a dramatic example of how inflammation is implicated in a number of interrelated health problems. In her case, chronic inflammation was associated with her high susceptibility to colds, infections, and bronchitis. I believe that inflammation was also responsible for the leptin resistance that slowly pushed Kate's weight to unacceptable levels.

If you, too, have wondered why those extra pounds you put on are so hard to take off; if, like Kate, you've noticed a slow but steady increase in your weight over the years; if you've got two or three sets of clothes, depending on where you are in your weight-loss cycle; or if you simply feel that maintaining your weight is a constant struggle, then you, too, are probably a victim of leptin resistance. Even if excess weight is your only health problem, you are probably suffering from a silent form of inflammation in which leptin resistance is sabotaging your attempts at weight control. The good news is that by correcting inflammation, you can overcome leptin resistance. This in turn will restore your body's natural weight-loss mechanism, causing the pounds to drop away effortlessly.

Your Weight: A Self-Regulating System

The concept of leptin resistance marks a major advance in our understanding of weight gain and weight loss. Most of us, doctors and scientists included, have believed for a long time that body fat was simply an inert storehouse of unused calories. In that view, weight management was a simple matter—exercise more, eat less, and the pounds will drop; reverse the process, and your weight will rise. More recent dietary theories—low fat, low carb, Atkins, the Zone, and South Beach—vary the equation by blaming particular types of foods (fats or carbs), or by insisting on a particular proportion among foods (such as the Zone's 40:30:30 ratio for carbs, fats, and proteins) to achieve optimal weight loss.

But the latest weight-loss research suggests that all of these approaches miss the point. Fat is not an inert storehouse of calories. It is an active organ that produces its own hormones. In fact, *our fat regulates itself.* When we gain weight, our fat produces a hormone known as leptin that suppresses our appetite and speeds up our metabolism, causing us to lose the extra pounds we've just put on. At least, that's how it's supposed to work. If this process fails to operate, then our fat-regulating hormones aren't working properly and we suffer from the hormonal imbalance known as leptin resistance.[2]

I'll say it again because I doubt you've ever heard it before: your fat is designed to regulate itself. When all your hormonal systems are functioning properly, you may gain a few pounds, but you will then lose them automatically.

The basis for this remarkable statement comes from one of the most exciting scientific breakthroughs to be made in recent years. In 1994, Jeffrey Friedman and his colleagues at Rockefeller University discovered leptin, a hormone whose main role is to let the brain know how much body fat you have.[3] If your body fat falls to a dangerously low level, leptin levels signal the brain to go into a state of emergency.[4] Fertility is one of the first casualties.[5] A woman with too little body fat can't ovulate or menstruate, because her body recognizes that she doesn't have enough fat to sustain a pregnancy or nurse a child. Leptin is a key messenger to convey this vital information.

On the other hand, if your body fat goes up past a certain point, what happens? Increased leptin levels signal your brain to suppress your appetite and speed up your metabolism.[6] Leptin actually increases your resting metabolic rate—the rate at which your body burns calories when it is at rest.[7] Clearly, a higher resting metabolic rate is another useful factor that can help us lose weight. And all of these beneficial effects result from a hormone that is produced by our own body fat.

Scientists' initial response to the discovery of leptin was to hope that human obesity was due to leptin deficiency, in the same way that childhood diabetes is due to a deficiency of insulin. What scientists discovered, however, was that overweight people have *high* levels of leptin—but their leptin isn't working properly. This condition has been labeled *leptin resistance*, and it has been compared to the insulin resistance (rather than insulin deficiency) that occurs in adult-onset diabetes. In leptin resistance, as in insulin resistance, there's nothing wrong with the hormone itself. The problem is that cells of your body cannot respond properly to the message the hormone is giving them.

The startling new understanding of body fat, which began

with the discovery of leptin resistance, will soon change our view of obesity forever. It demonstrates that if you are completely healthy, and if you have access to enough nutritious food, you can maintain a healthy weight naturally, without having to think about it.

Unfortunately, most Americans are simply not this healthy. Thanks to improper diet, lack of exercise, excessive stress, and exposure to environmental toxins—the very hallmarks of modern life—our bodies are not regulating weight properly. It's not only that certain types of fats, sugar, and red meat are fattening, but they also contribute to weight gain through their promotion of inflammation. And inflammation plays a direct role in triggering leptin resistance. By disrupting our body's natural weight-maintenance mechanisms, leptin resistance leads us to gain even more weight.

The key to easy, permanent weight loss, therefore, is to correct the leptin resistance that causes our weight to rise. Once we've cured leptin resistance—a cure that requires eliminating some foods from our diet and adding others—our bodies will maintain a healthy weight of their own accord.

I made this important discovery in two ways. First, as I described in Chapter 1, I developed early versions of the Fat Resistance Diet while trying to help my patients suffering from asthma, arthritis, colitis, skin problems, and certain cardiovascular problems, all triggered by inflammation. As patients followed my anti-inflammation diet, their inflammation subsided—and their weight dropped. This occurred time and time again with overweight patients, even if the patient had no specific interest in weight loss. Thus, before anyone had diagnosed the condition of leptin resistance, I was curing it by prescribing healthy, anti-inflammatory foods.

Second, I followed the latest scientific research on inflammation and obesity. Over time, the articles I read in scientific journals began to illuminate the relationship between the inflammation I was trying to cure and the obesity from which many of my patients suffered. As scientists advanced their discoveries, their findings helped to explain what I had already noticed: cure a person's inflammation through nutrition, and his or her weight will drop.

The final piece of the puzzle involved leptin resistance, which helped explain the deeper reasons why healing inflammation might help people restore and maintain a healthy weight. Once I understood the chain reaction—inflammation eventually led to leptin resistance, which in turn sabotaged weight-loss efforts—I understood that an anti-inflammatory diet could reverse the process and lead to permanent weight loss.

Now, if you think you've learned enough science for one day, feel free to skip ahead to Chapter 6 and start following the principles of the Fat Resistance Diet. You can successfully use the program I've outlined there without knowing anything more. But if you'd like to understand why the Fat Resistance Diet works so well and why it addresses so many health problems beyond obesity, read on. It's a fascinating story.

Inflammation: Self-Healing Gone Awry

Inflammation is your body's biochemical response to an assault. If you are bruised, injured, or attacked by a bacterial infection, chemicals in the affected tissue known as *cytokines* (cell movers) call for white blood cells to rush to the area and defend your body much as a dispatcher calls for an ambulance. The sudden influx of white blood cells and the related increase in blood flow is intended to be a healing response. But this process can sometimes be accompanied by uncomfortable side effects: the familiar redness, swelling, heat, fever, and pain that are considered the classic hallmarks of inflammation. Sometimes, these white blood cells arrive silently, without apparent symptoms, responding to toxins and infections of which we aren't even aware. But whether we know it or not, white cells congregate whenever cytokines put out their chemical call.

ADIPONECTIN: ANOTHER FAT-REGULATING HORMONE

Leptin isn't the only hormone that your fat produces. Another key player in the fat-regulation system is *adiponectin.* We're just beginning to understand this fascinating hormone, but we do know that it, like leptin, is produced only by the fat cells. Paradoxically, the more fat you have, the less adiponectin your fat cells produce.[8] Thus, higher levels of adiponectin are associated with a lower percentage of body fat—and lower weight.

High levels of adiponectin have all sorts of beneficial effects.[9] They help your muscles turn fat into energy more efficiently.[10] They fight inflammation.[11] They help increase insulin sensitivity, which in turn aids in the prevention of diabetes. Adiponectin also appears to protect the blood vessels, preventing hypertension and heart disease. And finally, like leptin, adiponectin suppresses appetite.

Remember, adiponectin is in short supply when you're overweight, so simply by losing excess weight, you can boost your stores of this key hormone. Now, instead of a vicious cycle, you've got a system of positive reinforcement: the more weight you lose, the more adiponectin you have—and the extra adiponectin helps you lose even more weight.[12]

There's another way to boost your adiponectin levels—by eating the right foods. Anthocyanins—pigments found in foods with deep red, blue, and purple colors, such as blueberries, cherries, blackberries, raspberries, and blue corn—support your body's production of this weight-loss-friendly hormone.[13] That's why the Fat Resistance Diet is rich in cherries and berries, which will both satisfy your palate and help you recover your hormonal balance. Who knew that eating sweet, delicious fruits could actually help you lose weight?

Of course, you wouldn't want a dispatcher to keep sending ambulances to the site after the problem had been solved. And you don't want your body to continue indefinitely with its inflammatory cries for help, particularly not when the healing effects of inflammation are so often accompanied by damage to our cells and organs—the swollen painful joints found in arthritis; the overly sensitive lungs that result from asthma; a variety of cardiovascular problems, including an increased risk of heart disease and stroke.[14] You might think of these negative side effects as the risk you take whenever you call an ambulance—along with the healing comes noise, confusion, and interruption of traffic. If you need the inflammation to heal an injury, the side effects are well worth the risk. But you don't want to invoke this chemical process any more often than you need to—and you want to turn it off as soon as you can.

Fortunately, our bodies are designed to offer a counter-response, a flood of anti-inflammatory chemicals that is triggered by the inflammation itself.[15] Think of these anti-inflammatory chemicals as the person standing behind the dispatcher. When the time is right, he'll say, "Stop calling for more ambulances and start sending those rescue vehicles back to headquarters. Everything is fine now, and we need to calm things down."

If inflammation is the "on" switch, the anti-inflammatory chemicals are the "off" switch. And since inflammation itself calls forth the anti-inflammatory chemicals, turning inflammation *on* leads directly to the chemical reaction that eventually turns inflammation *off*. In scientific terminology, this is known as a "negative feedback loop"—a process that is designed to shut itself down. It's like saying that our ambulance dispatcher, as soon as he arrives at work, puts in a call for the guy standing behind him, the one who will tell him when to send the ambulances back to base. Whenever the "inflammatory" dispatcher does his job, his "anti-inflammatory" counterpart waits nearby, ready to tell him when to stop.

This was a remarkably effective healing system in premodern times. Most of our inflammatory responses came as a result of infection or injury, known as *acute* inflammation—specifically triggered by an assault and damped down as quickly as possible by the anti-inflammatory response. The ambulance, so to speak, was called only for a true emergency, and it got sent back to base relatively soon. Perhaps the inflammatory response had some unpleasant side effects, but these were inconsequential compared to the urgency of healing the wound or infection.

Modern life, however, has produced a relatively new condition known as *chronic* or *silent* inflammation,[16] which can be caused by poor diet,[17] lack of exercise,[18] poorly managed stress,[19] environmental toxins[20]—and obesity.[21] Each of these factors represents a kind of low-grade assault on the body, and each one triggers an inflammatory response. Because this response is relatively small, we don't experience the more visible signs of inflammation—the swelling, pain, redness, and fever that come with an acute assault. But because the danger persists over weeks, months, and even years, our inflammatory response becomes continual. It's as if the ambulance is perpetually being called: instead of flaring up, solving the problem, and then disappearing, the inflammatory chemicals are continually being produced by our cells and then remaining within our bloodstream. If you're eating the wrong kinds of fats, consuming too much sugar, not getting enough exercise, mismanaging your stress, and carrying a significant amount of extra weight, you are creating a chronic state of low-grade inflammation.

This alone can cause all sorts of health problems, such as Kate's ongoing respiratory troubles. But according to some researchers, chronic, low-grade inflammation is also associated with more severe problems, including heart disease, cardiovascular problems, artherosclerosis, increased risk of stroke, and even cancer. Healing the inflammatory response in order to help people with these conditions has been a major part of my medical practice for the past three decades.

There's yet another problem with chronic inflammation, and this is the key to understanding leptin resistance. The continuous presence of inflammatory chemicals in the bloodstream calls forth the continuous production of anti-inflammatory chemicals as well. So here's where the story gets even more interesting.

One of the effects of some anti-inflammatory chemicals is to disrupt your body's response to leptin.

As we've seen, your fat produces leptin in order to regulate itself. Increased leptin levels should suppress your appetite and speed up your metabolism. But if you've got chronic inflammation, you'll also produce extra-high levels of *anti*-inflammatory chemicals. And these potentially helpful chemicals have one very negative effect: they trigger leptin resistance.

Leptin resistance prevents this crucial hormone from fulfilling its functions. Even if you've got very high levels of leptin—and the more body fat you have, the higher your levels will be—your leptin won't be doing its job, which is to suppress your appetite and boost your metabolism. As a result, you gain weight.

Fortunately, leptin resistance can be reversed, enabling you to lose weight. When I started treating patients like Kate with a diet designed to heal their inflammation, they began losing weight almost automatically. That's because, as their inflammation subsided, so did the levels of *anti*-inflammatory chemicals in their cells. And as these chemicals decreased, my patients' sensitivity to leptin returned. Suddenly, they were now able to respond to leptin's regulatory power, their appetite and metabolism working together to help them achieve a healthy weight.

How Obesity Creates Inflammation

Obesity itself is a direct cause of inflammation, in at least two major ways. First, some of the hormones produced by fat cells (called *adipokines*) set off your body's inflammatory response. The more body fat you have, the more inflammatory adipokines you will produce, particularly TNF-alpha (*tumor necrosis factor alpha*) and IL-6 (*interleukin-6*), which are produced by fat cells as well as by cells of the immune system. TNF is known for producing the tissue damage and pain associated with rheumatoid arthritis and other autoimmune conditions. It can also interfere with the operation of insulin and is a major contributor to insulin resistance.[22] (For more about insulin resistance, see Chapter 5.) IL-6 is closely related to TNF and is associated with arthritis and heart disease.

Second, fat tends to attract a type of white blood cell known as a *macrophage*, which also produces inflammatory chemicals.[23] Macrophages are scavenger cells, sometimes called the garbage collectors of the immune system, because their job is literally to gobble up cellular debris. These scavengers seem to be drawn to body fat because fat cells—especially if you're obese—tend to leak and break open. Macrophages move into the leaky fat tissue in order to clean up the mess. If that's all they did, we wouldn't have a problem. But once embedded in your fat, macrophages begin spewing out inflammatory chemicals—most notably, the pro-inflammatory cytokines TNF-alpha and IL-6.

Whenever a pro-inflammatory cytokine enters a cell, the cell releases a key group of anti-inflammatory chemicals called SOCS: *suppressors of cytokine signaling*. As their name suggests, SOCS molecules suppress inflammatory cytokines—but they also interfere with leptin.[24] Instead of allowing that hormone to suppress appetite and speed up metabolism, SOCS molecules disable that signal. Leptin resistance occurs and leads to weight gain. Indeed, leptin resistance is such a significant factor in weight gain that a recent Swedish study found that leptin-resistant men in a weight-loss program actually *gained* weight over the course of the study, even as their fellow participants were able to slim down.[25]

Leptin resistance is part of a true vicious cycle. Extra fat produces chronic, low-grade inflammation. The chronic inflammation produces a chronic *anti*-inflammatory response from your SOCS molecules. The SOCS response stops leptin from controlling your weight. So your weight goes up, which causes more inflammation. And the cycle starts all over again.

For each particular person, the cycle can start in a different way. If you've gained a lot of extra weight, that's one starting point. If you have a high intake of inflammatory foods—the wrong kinds of fat; refined sugar; red meat—that's another possible trigger. Depriving yourself of healing foods—omega-3 essential fatty acids, fiber, and antioxidants—is a third possibility. And mismanaged stress, toxic exposure, and insufficient exercise can be triggers as well.[26]

However this cycle of leptin resistance started, there's one simple way to stop it. Start eating according to the Fat Resistance Diet and follow the principles in Chapters 7, 8, and 9 with regard to exercise, stress, and toxins. Healing your inflammation will lower your anti-inflammatory chemicals, reducing the SOCS molecules and allowing leptin to do its job of regulating your weight. You will heal your leptin resistance and restore your body to its natural ability to regulate your weight.

Measuring Inflammation

As we've learned more about inflammation in recent years, we've also become more sophisticated at measuring it. One indicator in particular, C-reactive protein (CRP), has received attention as a useful marker of the level of inflammatory chemicals in your bloodstream. CRP appears to be a good indicator of the level of IL-6, a major inflammatory chemical. Obesity and weight gain are associated with a modest elevation of CRP, while, as we saw with Kate at the beginning of this chapter, weight loss produces a drop in CRP levels.

Elevated CRP levels are also associated with risk factors for many obesity-related disorders. If you have normal blood pressure, for example, but high CRP levels, that seems to be a good predictor of the future development of high blood pressure—suggesting that inflammation may be part of what causes your blood pressure to rise.[27] CRP levels are also beginning to be seen as a risk factor for coronary heart disease.[28] In aging adults, high CRP levels are associated with muscle weakness and frailty, suggesting that many of the effects we attribute to aging are actually the result of chronic inflammation, not age.[29] This further suggests that by following the Fat Resistance Diet, you can actually counter and even reverse some aspects of the aging process.

I myself have often measured the CRP levels of my obese patients before and after they began the Fat Resistance Diet. The results have been consistent: if CRP has been high, there is a marked drop after patients start to lose significant amounts of weight. Of course, CRP levels are likely to decline when any overweight person slims down, no matter what diet is used.[30] But the important news for people on the Fat Resistance Diet is this: *The steadier and more consistent the drop in CRP, the more likely you are to keep the weight off.* I have noticed this result in my patients repeatedly, and I am confident of the reason: Because the Fat Resistance Diet is carefully designed to heal low-grade chronic inflammation, it attacks the problem at its root. Once the inflammation is healed, leptin resistance is cured as well, and patients are able to maintain a healthy weight virtually without effort.

JONATHAN'S KITCHEN TIPS:

CHERRIES

As a reward for making it through the most challenging chapter in the book, we want to share a very special treat: cherries. Fresh in season, frozen, or as juice, we enjoy the delicious flavor and amazing health benefits of cherries throughout the year. To understand our passion for this sweet and tart fruit, just picture Dr. Galland looking in the freezer to find the organic cherries!

Studies on cherries reveal exciting results. Of central importance to losing weight, cherries have been shown to help lower CRP and inflammation. That's why our diet starts with a "cherry festival" of desserts on Days 2 and 12 of the Stage 1 meal plan. Enjoy!

Although I've used the Fat Resistance Diet to help my patients, I haven't yet been able to do a clinical study of it. But I have seen a clinical evaluation of a diet very similar to mine, published in the *Journal of the American Medical Association*.[31] The results of this study go a long way toward proving the extraordinary value of the Fat Resistance Diet.

The trial was conducted at the Division of Metabolic Diseases at the Second University of Naples in Italy. One hundred and twenty women were included in the randomized trial. Half were put on a "Mediterranean-style" diet, which, like the Fat Resistance Diet, is rich in fruits, vegetables, and omega-3 fats. The other half were put on a "prudent diet" of the kind recommended by the American Heart Association. Significantly, neither plan was intended to be a weight-loss diet. In fact, both plans supplied over 2,000 calories a day, which is a bit more than the average American woman consumes each day.

At the end of the study, both groups of women had lost weight. But the women on the Mediterranean diet had lost significantly more weight and body mass than those on the "prudent diet." Even more important, they had significant reductions in two key markers of bodywide inflammation: their levels of CRP and IL-6.

Furthermore, the women also saw a marked rise in their adiponectin levels, which, as described earlier in this chapter, contributes to continued weight loss, helps prevent diabetes, and improves cardiovascular health. Finally, the women experienced a measurable improvement in their insulin sensitivity. (For the relationship between insulin sensitivity, weight, and the Fat Resistance Diet, see Chapter 6.) While the scientists didn't measure the women's leptin sensitivity, every other result in this remarkable trial suggests that the women on this diet had overcome their leptin resistance and could look forward to continued weight loss and the long-term maintenance of a healthy weight.

LATEST RESEARCH FURTHER CONFIRMS THE SCIENCE OF THE FAT RESISTANCE DIET

Since publication of the first edition of *The Fat Resistance Diet*, exciting new research has further confirmed our theory that chronic inflammation leads to leptin resistance and causes weight gain. Research conducted in the United States, Italy, Spain, and Japan has shown a strong correlation between high blood levels of CRP (indicating inflammation) and high leptin levels (indicating leptin resistance).[32][33][34][35] The initial research did not indicate which came first—high CRP or high leptin. Then, in 2006, scientists at the University of Pittsburgh in Pennsylvania found that CRP directly binds to leptin and prevents it from entering cells.[36] They demonstrated clearly and directly that inflammation and CRP itself are a cause of leptin resistance.

More proof that chronic inflammation causes leptin resistance comes from a study of AMPK, an enzyme that acts as your body's main metabolic switch. AMPK (which stands for "adenosine monophosphate kinase") detects how much energy is stored in your body's cells for performing normal metabolic functions. When cellular energy is low, AMPK turns on and directs your cells to start making energy by burning up fat and sugar. The activation of AMPK in muscle and fat is absolutely essential for you to lose weight or have energy for exercise. In the brain, AMPK increases appetite, causing you to consume more food as fuel. Leptin is your body's chief hormonal regulator of AMPK. Leptin stimulates AMPK in fat and muscle and inhibits it in the brain, the perfect balance of effects for natural weight loss. A brilliant series of studies at the University of Melbourne in Australia has recently revealed that chronic inflammation impairs the ability of leptin to stimulate AMPK in human muscles.[37] The culprit? SOCS-3, the inflammation-induced protein that Harvard researchers have identified as the major cause of leptin resistance.[38]

This new research is so strong and consistent, we predict that in another 10 years the principles underlying the Fat Resistance Diet will be recognized by all physicians as the best approach to reversing the global obesity epidemic.

This has been the experience of my patients—including Kate, whom I recently saw for her five-year checkup. Happily slim and active, enjoying a healthy immune system, and savoring the many delicious food choices available to her, she clearly demonstrates the effectiveness of the Fat Resistance Diet and the healing power of food.

Summary of Chapter Two:
Leptin Resistance: The Reason You Can't Lose Weight

1. When we are healthy, our body fat regulates itself and weight loss is automatic.
2. Chronic inflammation caused by improper diet, excessive stress, and lack of physical activity causes leptin resistance. This interferes with the body's fat regulation.
3. Inflammation contributes to problems such as heart disease, increased risk of stroke, and cancer.
4. Healing the inflammation reverses leptin resistance. This enables weight loss and promotes well-being.

three

The Real Truth About Fats

first met my patient Beth in 1994. A fifty-three-year-old high school teacher, she came to me because of the joint pain that had been bothering her since she'd begun perimenopause, the transitional period that precedes menopause. But she was also worried about the twenty pounds she'd gained over the past two years.

"I don't understand it," she told me. "I've known for a long time that I have an allergy to wheat and corn, so I've cut those foods out of my diet. And I'm on a low-carb, high-protein diet—shouldn't that keep the weight off?"

Beth was especially concerned because she knew that many women tend to gain weight once menopause begins. "If I've gained this much now, what will I look like in five years?" she asked.

I'd been aware for some time that food allergies sometimes produce a variety of symptoms, including the prevention of weight loss. For some people, food allergies seem to produce fluid retention, causing them to bloat and swell. Beth had been one of these people, and after working with a doctor when she was in her early thirties, she'd identified her allergens and cut them out of her diet. Soon after, the headaches that had plagued her went away. Her swollen hands and feet returned to normal. And she lost the ten pounds she'd gained.

Then, soon after turning fifty, she'd started gaining weight once again, accompanied by pain in her joints, hands, elbows, wrists, hips, and knees. Specialists had ruled out arthritis, lupus, and a thyroid condition, and her internist had told her that both the weight gain and joint pain were common among peri-menopausal women. He'd suggested estrogen, but that only added swollen, achy breasts to her list of symptoms. That's when she came to me.

"Let's look at your diet," I suggested.

"I eat in a very healthy way," she insisted. "In fact, I'm prac-tically on the Atkins diet—and I'm very strict about portion sizes. I'm sure I'm not allergic to anything I'm eating—by now, believe me, I know my symptoms." Beth went on to point out that she was consuming only about 1,600 to 1,800 calories each day—slightly less than the average American woman.

But when Beth finished telling me about her weekly food in-take, I knew we'd found the problem. Despite her attempts at healthy eating, about 40 percent of the calories in her diet came from fat, particularly saturated fats and trans fats, two types of fat that are known to produce inflammation. At the same time, she was getting almost no omega-3 fat, a type of anti-inflammatory fat that is essential to the healthy functioning of both body and brain.

"So you've got two problems," I informed her. "One is that it's almost impossible to eat a high-protein, low-carb diet without also consuming large amounts of fat. You've got to shift the ra-tios a bit, consuming more carbs so that you can eat less fat."

"That's the exact opposite of low carb," Beth protested.

"It's not about carbohydrates," I said. "Our bodies need lots of fresh fruits and vegetables. To stay healthy, you need nine serv-ings of fruits and vegetables each day. You can't eat like that on a low-carb diet—but those are the foods you need."

Beth nodded. "What's the other problem?" she asked.

"It's not just a question of eating less fat. You've actually got to eat *more* of certain kinds of fats—the omega-3s that can help you fight inflammation."

By the time I met Beth, I had been using omega-3 fats in my medical practice for more than fifteen years, and had been teaching other doctors about them for more than a decade. A number of studies published in the late 1980s and early 1990s showed that people with rheumatoid arthritis—a disease produced by excessive inflammation—could significantly relieve their symptoms by consuming fish oil supplements, which are rich in omega-3s.[1] Beth was familiar with this research, because it had received considerable media attention.

"So I need to take fish oil supplements, or eat more salmon, is that what you're saying?"

"Not exactly," I replied. "The studies I've seen show that people with rheumatoid arthritis—whose symptoms resemble yours—need at least 2.5 grams of supplemental omega-3 fatty acids each day to make a difference. To get that from food, you'd need to eat an 8-ounce salmon steak each day—not impossible, but a bit limiting. However, if you reduce your intake of other types of fats—cutting back on meat, egg yolks, whole-fat dairy products, and vegetable oil—you actually don't need as much omega-3 to produce the same effect. In other words, there are two issues with fat: how much you're consuming, and the proportions of each type."

Together, Beth and I worked out an alternative diet for her. She drastically reduced her consumption of meat and butter, and cut out the French fries that were her main deviation from her low-carb regimen. She avoided any foods made with trans fats—those fats found in partially hydrogenated vegetable oils, and thus in virtually all packaged or processed foods. And she ate more fish, flaxseeds, and walnuts, all rich in omega-3 essential fatty acids.

The results were dramatic. Within a few weeks, her joint pain was almost gone—and without even trying, she lost ten pounds over the next two months. Simply by paying attention to her fat consumption, Beth continued to lose the rest of the weight she'd put on, and she's managed to keep it off for the past ten years. When she did go through menopause, she was symptom-free, which I attribute to her anti-inflammatory diet. And her cholesterol, which had been slowly climbing before she saw me, is now lower than at any time she can remember.

Most satisfying for me, however, was the comment Beth made when I saw her again last month, a remark that I've heard echoed by many patients over the years. "The best thing about this way of eating is that I really don't have to think about it," she told me. "I'm so used to eating this way, my body knows what it needs, and I just eat whatever I'm hungry for. I feel great, and I never gain weight—what more can you ask for?"

Breaking Through the Myths About Fat

After the low-fat diet craze of the 1980s and the low-carb mania of the 1990s, most Americans are left with two conflicting myths about fat:

MYTH #1: Fat is bad for you, and a healthy diet involves eating as little fat as possible.

MYTH #2: Fats aren't the problem—carbs are. So you can eat as much fat as you want, as long as you're cutting back on the carbs.

These myths have alternated over the years, with first one, then the other dominating the popular understanding of nutrition. But as early as twenty years ago, in my book *Superimmunity for Kids*, I argued against both. So let's take a closer look at what's wrong with each of these propositions.

MYTH #1: Fat is bad for you, and a healthy diet involves eating as little fat as possible.

Nathan Pritikin has been one of the best-known proponents of this misconception. It's true that *some* types of fat are extremely bad for you—particularly trans fats, which, as I've said, are found in hydrogenated vegetable oils and in virtually all packaged and processed foods. Frankly, I'd be happy to see you cut all trans fats out of your diet, period.

But some other types of fats are not only good for you, they are essential to the healthy functioning of your body and your brain. And still other types of fats, while not essential, are not particularly harmful and will help make your food tastier and more satisfying. Also, a moderate amount of fat in the diet helps you digest and absorb fat-soluble nutrients, including carotenoids, vitamin A, and vitamin E. *The trick is to eat the right fats in the right proportions.*

MYTH #2: Fats aren't the problem—carbs are. So you can eat as much fat as you want, as long as you're cutting back on the carbs.

This myth grew out of the Atkins diet. For many Americans, it's hard to imagine a more attractive proposition than to be told that they can eat all the steak, bacon, and eggs they like. But it's just not a healthy approach to eating.

First, many types of fat are inflammatory. Saturated fat, for example—a type of fat found primarily in meat, poultry, and dairy products—has powerful direct and indirect pro-inflammatory effects that can be measured after only a single meal. We can also correlate levels of inflammation with the over-all level of saturated fat in a person's diet.[2] Significantly, you can suffer from fat-related inflammation without necessarily having symptoms—though, like Beth, many people do experience heart-burn, bloating, fatigue, and acne, in addition to joint and muscle pain, on a high-fat diet. In some cases, these symptoms clear up on a low-carb diet—but as long as you're eating large amounts of saturated fat, your inflammation will persist, whether or not your symptoms do. So don't be fooled. Eating a diet high in saturated fat virtually guarantees that you will suffer from inflammation as well as the leptin resistance and obesity that result.

Second, fats are very calorie-dense. Whereas proteins and carbs contain about 4 calories per gram, fats contain 9 calories. So the low-carb approach is right about one thing: if you're going to lose or maintain weight on a high-fat diet, you've got to cut way back on the carbs; otherwise, you'll be eating way too many calories. But cutting out nuts and seeds, fruits, beans, and starchy vegetables means that you're depriving yourself of fiber and many vitamins, minerals, and other nutrients that your body desperately needs to stay healthy. The moment you get tired of eating such a restricted diet and add some carbs back into your daily intake, the combination of carbs and high-calorie fat will cause you to gain back any weight you lost on the more restricted aspects of the plan. Meanwhile, all the bad fats you've eaten—such as those found in meat, bacon, butter, and cream—have inflamed your body, setting you up for the leptin resistance that will make future weight loss and weight maintenance very difficult. Again, *the trick is to eat the right fats in the right proportions.*

I know it's hard to believe that the dietary advice that has gained so much popularity is simply wrong. But as a scientist and a doctor, I assure you that it is. Let me tell you two basic principles on which I constructed the Fat Resistance Diet:

1. NO trans fats of any kind.
2. A weekly fat intake that constitutes between 25 and 30 percent of the total calories in your diet, in roughly the following proportions:

   • No more than one-third saturated fats. The saturated fat naturally found in lean meat, poultry, low-fat dairy products, seafood, and some vegetables will readily fill this quota. Avoid less healthy saturated fat sources like butter, cream, margarine, and shortening.

- About one-third monounsaturated fats. These are found in olive oil, many nuts and seeds, and other healthy, traditional vegetable oils.
- About one-third polyunsaturated fats. You can get these from eating fish and certain nuts and seeds and their oils. Of these polyunsaturated fats, roughly one-fifth should be omega-3s.

Essential Fats: Your Weight-Loss Allies

I've just told you what you need to know about how to choose a healthy balance of fats for your weight-loss and weight-maintenance diets. And of course, if you follow the meal plans and recipes in Part Three, you'll automatically be eating according to these guidelines. But if you'd like to know a bit more about why the right balance of fat is so important, read on.

Most of the fat we eat—and the fat in our bodies—is composed of fatty acids. Basically, a fatty acid is a string of carbon atoms with a specially arranged pair of oxygen atoms at one end. The carbon atoms are bonded either to each other or to hydrogen atoms. If all the possible spaces on all the carbon atoms are filled with hydrogen, the fat is *saturated*—literally, saturated with hydrogen. If hydrogen atoms are missing, the fat is *unsaturated*.

Without the bonding effect of hydrogen, carbon atoms become unstable. So, in unsaturated fats, the carbon atoms create extra bonds with each other, called double bonds. If a fat molecule has only one double bond, it's known as *monounsaturated fat. (Mono* means "one.") If a fat molecule has more than one double bond, it's known as *polyunsaturated fat. (Poly*, of course, means "many.")

As it happens, the body can make its own saturated and monounsaturated fat from the carbohydrates you consume. But the

GET TO KNOW YOUR FATS, PART 1

TRANS FATS—FATS TO AVOID

My advice on trans fats is very simple: don't eat them. They're extremely bad for your health—and they interfere with weight loss as well, as you'll see later in this chapter.

SOURCES: Any food made with hydrogenated or partially hydrogenated vegetable oil, which may include biscuits, cakes, cinnamon rolls, cookies, corn chips, potato chips, crackers, doughnuts, commercial granola, frozen desserts, muffins, pastries, pies, commercial popcorn, shortening, and mayonnaise.

NOTE: The "No Trans Fats" label now appearing on many prepared foods can be misleading. Federal law allows "No Trans Fats" to apply to any food with less than half a gram of trans fats per serving. By making the official serving size small enough, manufacturers can label foods made with hydrogenated oils as having "No Trans Fat."

SATURATED FATS—UP TO ONE-THIRD OF YOUR FAT INTAKE

If you eat lean meat and some seafood, you'll be filling your quota of saturated fats. Avoid butter, cream, margarine, and shortening. If you consume high-fat animal foods such as these, or bacon or chicken skin, you will easily overdose on saturated fats, which will tend to promote weight gain, inflammation, and cardiovascular problems.

ANIMAL SOURCES: Beef/pork/lamb/bacon; dairy products; poultry skin.

NOTE: Fish and shellfish may contain saturated fats, but significantly less than the amount of unsaturated fat.

PLANT SOURCES: Coconut oil, palm kernel oil, avocado.

(Continued)

MONOUNSATURATED FATS—UP TO ONE-THIRD OF YOUR FAT INTAKE

You need a moderate amount of these friendly fats to help you digest and absorb anti-inflammatory nutrients, many of which are fat-soluble. You can get some of the fat you need from omega-3 sources, too, but you can't eat enough omega-3 food sources to get all the fat you need, and other types of fats are pro-inflammatory. Monounsaturated fats appear to be beneficial. Their consumption is associated with a decreased rate of heart disease and related problems.

SOURCES: Olives, olive oil, almonds/almond oil, sesame seeds, pumpkin seeds, cashews, macadamia nuts, hazelnuts (filberts), pistachios, pine nuts, and avocados are your best bets.

NOTE: Peanuts contain equal amounts of monounsaturated and omega-6 polyunsaturated fats, but I don't recommend peanuts or peanut oil in the Fat Resistance Diet because peanuts tend to be contaminated with mold-derived toxins.

NOTE: Poultry and fish contain both monounsaturated and saturated fats but tend to have more monounsaturates than saturates.

POLYUNSATURATED FATS—AT LEAST ONE-THIRD OF YOUR FAT INTAKE

There are two types of polyunsaturated fats: omega-3s and omega-6s. (I'll explain the difference later in this chapter.) The amount of omega-3 fat you need is partly determined by how much omega-6 fat you consume. Ideally, your ratio of omega-6s to omega-3s should be 4:1, so make sure you're eating at least one-fourth as much omega-3 fat as omega-6 fat. However, the more omega-3 fats you consume relative to omega-6 fats, the better.

OMEGA-3s

FISH SOURCES: Fish, especially anchovy, bluefish, herring (pickled, not creamed), mackerel (Atlantic is the only safe kind), sablefish, salmon, sardines (fresh or canned in their own oil), sturgeon, and tuna (fresh is better; bluefin, not albacore). Conch is the one shellfish high in omega-3s.

VEGETABLE SOURCES: Flaxseeds and flaxseed oil.

NOTE: Other sources of omega-3s are walnuts and walnut oil, soybeans, and navy and kidney beans. You can get some omega-3s from green leafy vegetables of all types, but you need a lot of these because there's very little fat in them. Soybean oil contains a slight amount of omega-3s, but I don't recommend using it: it's very high in omega-6s as well, and the amount of omega-3s you get isn't worth it.

OMEGA-6s

SOURCES: Most vegetable oils: corn, safflower, sunflower, and soy oil; Brazil nuts; pumpkin seeds; sesame seeds and sesame oil.

NOTE: We use sesame seeds and sesame oil in the Fat Resistance Diet because they are rich in minerals and phytonutrients, impart delicious flavor to food, and contain as much monounsaturated fat as omega-6s— making them superior to other omega-6 sources.

body can't turn carbohydrates into the key polyunsaturated fats, even though it needs these essential fatty acids for a whole host of functions, including brain function, the regulation of immunity and hormone function, anti-inflammatory support,[3] and the creation of healthy skin and hair. In fact, almost nothing happens in your body that is not influenced by the polyunsaturated fatty acids in your cells.

When I explain this concept to patients, the first thing they want to know is, "How many essential fatty acids do I need each day?" And the answer is, "That depends."

Although there is a minimum absolute requirement for daily intake of essential fatty acids—about 4 percent of your total caloric intake—this requirement doesn't really mean much for most of us.[*] When our total fat intake goes up, we need to consume more essential fatty acids proportionally. That's because we need the essential fatty acids to counteract the inflammatory properties of other types of fats. So I'll say it again: *The trick is to eat the right fats in the right proportions.*

Now, there's one more distinction you need to know about: the two types of polyunsaturated fats. (These are summarized in the box "Get to Know Your Fats, Part 1.") Remember that, for the most part, polyunsaturated fats include the types of fatty acids your body can't produce by itself, making these essential fatty acids (EFAs). One type of EFA is omega-6; the other is omega-3. (The numbers refer to the location of the first double bond when you count down from the end of the carbon chain.) You need both omega-6s and omega-3s in your diet because you cannot change one kind into another and they have different effects in the body, as I'll explain further on.

Omega-6 fatty acids are widely available in animal foods, including meat, chicken, fish, milk products, and eggs. If you eat these foods, you are not likely to become deficient in omega-6s. Omega-3s, by contrast, are produced by green plants, especially seaweed, grass, and leaves, but their concentration in these plant foods is low because green plants contain so little fat. Some plants concentrate omega-3s in their seeds, particularly flaxseeds (as it happens, the health food of the Romans). Walnuts, soybeans, navy beans, and kidney beans also have modest amounts of omega-3s—but they have even higher levels of omega-6s. So your best way to get omega-3s is probably through fish, especially oily cold-water fish like salmon, which consume the omega-3s found in sea algae. Similarly, wild game animals that graze on grass and leaves and accumulate very little body fat have a relatively high concentration of omega-3s in their flesh. For Stone Age hunters, wild game constituted a major source of omega-3s. In our modern world, however, it's more practical to depend on fish.

The optimum dietary ratio of omega-3s to omega-6s appears to vary depending on the individual and his or her state of health, although the average ideal ratio of omega-6s to omega-3s is probably about 4:1. Research, however, suggests that while a ratio of 4:1 improves the outcome of patients with heart disease; a ratio of 5:1 improves asthma; and a ratio of 2.5:1 is needed to improve rheumatoid arthritis.[5]

Compare any of these healthy goals to the average American ratio, which—thanks to our high consumption of vegetable oils and our low consumption of fish and leafy green vegetables—is about 20:1. This unbalanced omega-6 to omega-3 ratio is one of the major causes of our widespread epidemic of chronic, low-grade inflammation—which results, as we saw in Chapter 2, in leptin resistance and persistent obesity.

Understanding the Weight-Loss Power of Omegas

"So how will consuming omega-3 fats help me lose weight?" Beth wanted to know when I first brought the topic to her attention.

Actually, when Beth first asked the question, in 1994, I wasn't able to give her as complete or accurate an answer as I can provide now. Scientific understanding of the many roles played by omega-3 fats in the body has advanced considerably since the 1990s. In fact, we're just beginning to understand the many anti-inflammatory cellular effects of omega-3 fats.

You don't need much omega-3 fat to ensure that this nutrient accomplishes its essential tasks. Only about 1 percent of your to-tal calories needs to come from omega-3 fat, or about 1.5 to 2.5 grams a day. Still, if you don't fill your plate with leafy green vegetables *and* eat 12 or more ounces of fish or wild game a week, you are likely to fall short. You can easily make up for the shortfall with a tablespoon or two of ground flaxseeds, or a half cup of walnuts.

However—and here's the rub—this small amount of omega-3 is only enough *if you're not eating too much omega-6 fats*. Omega-6 fats compete with omega-3 fats for transport into cells and can crowd the omega-3s out of the way, taking their place in the body's metabolic processes and keeping the body from making use of them. The more omega-6s there are, the more omega-3s you need in order to offset the competition. That's why I keep stressing the importance of balancing the different types of fat you consume. It's not just how much fat you eat; the proportions of different types of fat are also highly important.

Luckily, it's not hard to balance fats properly once you know how. If you follow the principles laid out in Chapter 6, and the meal plans and recipes in Part Three, you'll be fine. And you'll soon see how easy—and delicious—it is to eat this way. As Beth discovered, once you get used to balancing your fats, your body will virtually do this on its own.

Unnatural Fats: Your Weight-Loss Enemies

As mentioned earlier, there is one type of fat you should cut from your diet completely: the artificial hydrogenated fat that contains trans fatty acids. Trans fatty acids are rarely found in nature, but they are common in the American diet. That's because industrial scientists discovered that polyunsaturated fat—which tends to go bad very quickly when it's not refrigerated—has a far longer shelf life when it has been infused with hydrogen.

Incomplete or partial hydrogenation produces polyunsaturated fatty acids that are relatively stiff and straight, like a saturated fatty acid, but which the body tries to treat as if they were unsaturated. This produces profound biochemical confusion in your body's cells, making trans fat the most dangerous type of

GET TO KNOW YOUR FATS, PART 2

It's easy to tell the different types of fat apart, once you know the secret. The more saturated a fat is—the more loaded down with hydrogen molecules—the more heat is required to melt it. Saturated fats
tend to be stiff and sturdy: butter, the fat you trim from a piece of meat,
even coconut oil, which resembles wax at room temperature. They will
melt eventually, but they require more heat than occurs at the usual
room temperature to change from solid to liquid.

Monounsaturated fats, by contrast, are liquid at room temperature,
though they tend to get thick and viscous when you refrigerate them. Think
of olive oil, for example, which flows easily at room temperature but hardens
in the fridge. The double bond keeps these fat molecules loose and flexible.

Polyunsaturated fats are made up of molecules that are even more
curved and wiggly. Safflower and fish oil, for example, are not only
liquid at room temperature, but also after refrigeration. Even when you
freeze them, it's hard to get them to turn solid.

fat there is. I started warning my patients to avoid foods made
with partially hydrogenated vegetable oils almost thirty years
ago, when I first started exploring the relationship between
fatty acids and health. The laboratory science made it clear that
trans fats interfere with the way the body utilizes essential fatty
acids. In other words, no matter how many healthy omega-3s
and omega-6s you consume, if you also consume trans fats, you
are undermining your own efforts at health (and, as always, sabotaging your weight loss).

Meanwhile, the food industry lobbied heavily in favor of
trans fats, and few scientists or nutritionists would condemn
them publicly. Finally, groundbreaking research from Dr. Walter
Willett at Harvard University and from several research centers
in Europe established a definite association between trans fat

GRASS-FED CATTLE, CORN-FED GAME, AND FARM-RAISED SALMON

In recent years, some of my patients have asked me whether grass-fed cattle are a good source of omega-3s. The answer is a qualified yes. Range-fed cattle have lower levels of saturated fat and higher levels of omega-3 fats in their meat than do grain-fed cattle. Australian scientists found that range-fed cattle have a high enough omega-3 content to meet their government's standards for "good" or "moderately good" omega-3 sources. Canadian researchers have found that bison, which like cattle are grazing ruminants, have an omega-6 to omega-3 ratio in their flesh that is close to 4:1. Wild game, like elk and deer, however, have even lower levels of saturated fat and even lower omega-6 to omega-3 ratios (as low as 2:1). But beware: more and more game meats are being raised domestically, fed corn or various types of grain-based cattle feed. Such meat does not contain the same fat as true wild game—even if it is labeled "organic."

Wild salmon is rich in omega-3s because wild fish feed on natural plant foods that are also rich in omega-3s. The omega-3 content of farm-raised salmon depends upon how they are fed. Research done in Australia and France indicates that properly farmed salmon actually has a higher omega-3 content than wild salmon.

consumption and the risk of heart disease, especially in women. In the famous Harvard Nurses' Study, trans fats were found to be about twice as dangerous as saturated fats.[6] Subsequent research showed that trans fats raise cholesterol to higher levels and promote inflammation, insulin resistance, and leptin resistance.[7] To make matters worse, a recent study discovered that trans fats tend to increase your waist size.[8] So as you can see, trans fats are very dangerous products that play no beneficial role whatsoever in human nutrition—and in fact, they prevent your body from getting the nutrients it needs. You should avoid them as much as possible.

Restoring a Healthy Relationship to Dietary Fats

The last time I saw Beth, she asked me a fascinating question. "Why," she wondered, "is it so difficult to balance our fat intake? How did people without doctors and nutritionists ever manage?"

As it happened, I had the answer to her question. According to research by anthropologists and epidemiologists who have analyzed the dietary habits of early humans, Stone Age humans consumed far more omega-3s than we do now, primarily from wild game, which fed on leaves and grasses. Most of the meat we consume today is fed on grain or other products.[9]

JONATHAN'S KITCHEN TIPS:
SKIM OR LOW-FAT DAIRY

Dairy is an excellent source of calcium and protein, but it can also be a source of unwanted saturated fat. That's why the recipes and meal plans in the Fat Resistance Diet use only nonfat or low-fat milk, cheese, and yogurt. These recipes grew out of our long experience using nonfat or low-fat dairy in our own kitchens. The goal is to keep the flavor and nutrition but lose the fat. For example, our dessert recipes benefit from sweet and tart fruit concentrates, crunchy walnuts and almonds, ripe fruit, and fresh mint. So what about butter for cooking, flavoring dishes, or spreading on bread? We switched to extra virgin olive oil many years ago and haven't looked back. Extra virgin olive oil has a rich, satisfying flavor that goes perfectly with salads and bread. Recent studies indicate that extra virgin olive oil helps fight inflammation, which makes it an important part of the Fat Resistance Diet. Enjoy!

So, I told Beth, our current dietary dilemma is relatively recent—the result of our increased consumption of beef as well as other other sources of the wrong fats, along with our decreased consumption of omega-3s. I believe that the change in fat consumption has had profound effects on human physiology and has contributed significantly to the epidemic of inflammation-related disease, particularly the growing worldwide prevalence of obesity. I don't think that human beings will ever return to the dietary habits of our Stone Age ancestors, but the Fat Resistance Diet can guide you in making food choices that will both protect your health and enable you to lose weight.

Summary of Chapter Three: The Real Truth About Fats

1. It is a myth that all fats are bad and cause weight gain.
2. In fact, healthy fats are weight-loss allies and necessary for well-being.
3. Our diet, rich in omega-3 fats from walnuts, salmon, and beans, helps heal inflammation and reverse leptin resistance.
4. Do not eat any trans fats. Skip any oil labeled hydrogenated or partially hydrogenated.

four

The Real Truth About Carbs

My patient Jake was known as the Barbecue King of Rockland County. A hard-driving lawyer in his early forties, Jake spoke of himself as someone who "works hard, plays hard, loves to eat, and loves to cook!" Throughout his teens and young adulthood he'd always been an athletic guy—a basketball player and pole-vaulter in high school and college, and a basketball player throughout his stint in law school.

But when Jake got married, moved to the suburbs, and had two kids, he stopped exercising—and started to gain weight. By the time he was in his late thirties, Jake had gained nearly fifty-five pounds—an increase that meant he was unable to play basketball without getting winded. His blood pressure, cholesterol, and triglycerides had all gone up, and his doctor had warned him that unless he lost a significant amount of weight, he'd end up on medication.

Jake was used to taking action to solve his problems, so he went straight to a nutritionist. She put Jake—a big man at six foot two and 230 pounds—on a diet of 1,800 calories per day, which should have produced a weight loss of about a pound a week. And it did—until Jake had lost fifteen pounds. Then he plateaued.

So Jake tried to solve the problem himself. He started choosing healthier foods for his barbecues—less meat, more seafood—and he switched from barbecue sauce to hot sauce, because hot sauce has less fat and Jake had heard that hot sauce could speed up his metabolism. He also added a big salad to every meal, garnished with low-fat dressing. And for a while, Jake's plan worked—until he plateaued again after losing another ten pounds.

"OK, Doc, I'm at the end of my rope," Jake told me bluntly. "I'm still thirty-five pounds overweight, and I feel like I've run out of options. I started working out for thirty minutes a day, three days a week—but I really don't have time for more. I've cut out everything I can think of—and I've got to tell you, I feel like I'm in a food prison. And the last straw is that now I'm getting pain and stiffness in my joints—hips, knees, feet, and shoulders—even if I go for a week or two without working out. What's going on?"

I reviewed Jake's diet—and I concluded that inflammation and leptin resistance were at the root of his problems. In Jake's case, it was a question of both what he was eating and what he was *not* eating. Although his new effort to eat more seafood meant that he actually was getting a decent amount of omega-3 fats into his weekly diet, he was falling short in the fruit and vegetable department. Although the National Academy of Sciences now recommends nine daily servings of vegetables and fruits, Jake was eating barely five per day, and these often came in the form of iceberg lettuce and cucumber, two of the least nutritious vegetables. I was also concerned about the amount of hot chili sauce he was using to spice up his food. I have seen patients with arthritis in whom chili peppers actually provoked inflammation (see the box "Hold the Chili Peppers, Please" on page 60), and I thought Jake might be having similar troubles.

Moreover, I thought Jake would benefit greatly from the anti-inflammatory properties of other herbs and spices—garlic, onions, ginger, turmeric, fresh parsley, and basil—that would both improve his health and brighten up his diet. Likewise, he could make good use of tart cherry concentrate and pomegranate juice, which can be used, among other things, to marinate meat. Not only would cherry and pomegranate juice make his meat more flavorful, they would combat the inflammatory properties of animal fat—helping Jake to heal his inflammation, overcome his leptin resistance, and, eventually, lose weight.

"Let's try an experiment," I proposed. "I want you to eat not just five servings of vegetables a day, but nine. And I want those nine to come from the most intensely flavored, brightly colored fruits and vegetables available. Their flavor and color are signs of healing properties that can make a significant difference in your inflammation, and eventually in your weight."[1]

"I don't know, Doc." I had seen the look on Jake's face before— the look of a man who thought he'd finally reached the age when no one would ever again tell him to eat his vegetables. "It's been hard enough adding a salad into my diet. I've never been much of a fruit and vegetable guy."

"Well, give it a try," I told him. "Berries are terrific—blueberries, strawberries, blackberries—eat some of those every day, and try adding some cherry concentrate or pomegranate juice to your barbecue sauce. Look for bright orange carrots, deep-green spinach, crimson tomatoes. I want you eating crucifers at least four times a week—broccoli, cabbage, kale, Brussels sprouts. And you should get some onions and garlic into your diet every day—the more, the better. Let's break you out of that food prison and cure your inflammation at the same time."

The Barbecue King was intrigued. He started using tart cherry concentrate and pomegranate juice in his sauces and spicing his grilled items with turmeric, ginger, basil, and garlic. I shared with him some of the recipes that my son Jonathan had been working on—the very same recipes you'll find in Part Three of this book. Jake took to these tasty food choices immediately, grilling sweet peppers, zucchini, and tomatoes beside his chicken kebabs and salmon steaks; freshening his meals with huge salads made of romaine lettuce, arugula, scallions, and parsley.

Within a few days, Jake's joint pains had diminished. And the exquisite flavors and sauces he was able to create with his new palette of anti-inflammatory herbs and spices revived his enthusiasm for cooking—and for eating. Busy as he was, the recipes were so easy and quick that once he had stocked his

HOLD THE CHILI PEPPERS, PLEASE

Before he came to me, Jake was seasoning almost every item in his "food prison" with hot chili peppers or Tabasco sauce. Instead of availing himself of the wide range of tastes and scents provided by anti-inflammatory spices, Jake was simply making his food hotter and hotter. In doing so, he may have been literally inflaming his system.

Studies from Latin America and India have shown that a high intake of chili peppers is associated with an increased rate of stomach and gallbladder cancer.[2] And laboratory studies have indicated that capsaicin, a chemical found in chili peppers, can actually trigger inflammation by activating a newly discovered type of cell receptor called the *vanilloid receptor*.[3] I have seen cases of people with arthritis who improved dramatically when they eliminated chili peppers from their diet.

I recommend you put hot chili peppers on hold for most of your diet plan, along with jalapeños. Instead, focus on developing a broader palette of tastes and scents with the spices listed in the box "Savory Spices" in Chapter 6 on page 101. If you must heat things up, try black pepper. The piperine in this all-purpose spice appears to enhance the absorption of *flavonoids*—the healing properties of brightly colored, intensely flavored foods—so that pepper actually enhances the anti-inflammatory effect of fruits and vegetables.[4]

pantry with the right ingredients, it took no more time than the way he'd always prepared food. The doors to his "food prison" had opened wide.

Meanwhile, Jake was starting to lose weight, slowly but surely. Over the next six months, he lost thirty-five pounds, making it down to his young-adult weight of 190. Both his blood pressure and his cholesterol declined—his blood pressure from 135/90 down to 118/70; his LDL cholesterol from 160 to 98. It's been about six months since I last saw him, but a recent phone call assured me that Jake had remained at his healthy weight—and was experimenting with still more savory sauces.

Carbs or Fat Resistance Foods?

Just as we've been assaulted with inaccurate and contradictory myths about fat, so have most of us been miseducated about carbohydrates. By the time you've read this section, I hope you'll agree with my own scientific opinion, one that has been reinforced by my patients' dietary success: *Although some carbs can interfere with weight loss and contribute to a wide variety of health problems, other carbohydrates are Fat Resistance Foods, supporting health, curing inflammation—and promoting weight loss.* (Some herbs, spices, and teas are Fat Resistance Foods, too, along with some fish and dairy products. For a complete listing of the Top 50 Fat Resistance Foods, see page 8 in Chapter 1.)[5]

First, let's define carbohydrates. They're a form of hydrated (watery) carbon: a combination of carbon, hydrogen, and oxygen. Animal foods, with the exception of milk, are almost devoid of carbohydrates. Virtually all our dietary carbohydrates come from plant foods: fruits, vegetables, nuts, seeds, and grains.

Now, let's demolish those misconceptions about carbs one by one, until only the truth is left standing.

MYTH #1: Carbohydrates can be divided into two categories: simple and complex. The simple carbs are bad for your health and weight; the complex carbs are good.

Well, at least part of that myth is true. Carbohydrates *can* be divided into simple and complex. All plant-based foods contain both simple and complex carbohydrates. Sugars are simple carbs—and they're abundant in sweet foods like honey, sugar cane (which is a grain), sweet corn (also a grain), beets, and most fruits. Starches are complex carbs; they're abundant in corn, wheat, and other grains and in potatoes.

Would it surprise you to realize that white flour—a food that most of us agree isn't particularly healthful or conducive to weight loss—actually contains complex carbohydrates? After all, it's a starchy food. True, the starch in white flour isn't particularly good for either your health or your weight, but it *is* complex—exactly as complex as the starch found in whole grains or unrefined flour. You can probably see why this distinction isn't very helpful as far as diet is concerned.

What *is* helpful is looking not at the carb, but at its package. Both white rice and brown rice contain complex carbs—starches rather than sugars. Yet a processed grain of white rice comes in a fiberless kernel with very few nutrients, while a natural grain of brown rice comes encased in fiber—a vital component of a healthy diet, as we'll soon see—along with B vitamins and other nutrients. It's not enough to look at the carb's complexity; you have to look at its package.

The same principle holds when comparing simple carbs (sugars) with complex carbs (starches). The simple carbs found in carrots and berries are both more nutritious and more supportive of weight loss than the complex carbs found in potatoes and flour. That's because the carbs in carrots and berries come in a package that's rich in nutrients—especially anti-inflammatory nutrients—while the potatoes and flour are relatively deficient in anti-inflammatory nutrients. I'd rather have my patients snacking on the simple carbs found in carrots and berries than on the complex carbs that occur in baked potatoes or a baguette.

When I explained this principle to Jake, he was a bit confused at first. "How can you tell which carbs are good for you?" he wanted to know.

To some extent, I told him, you just have to learn them. Start with my list of Top 50 Fat Resistance Foods and with the foods on the Fat Resistance Diet. By the time you've eaten this way for a few weeks, you'll know which fruits, vegetables, and grains have the highest nutrients.

You can also use color as a basic—though not infallible—rule of thumb. Generally, the most intensely colored fruits and vegetables are the most nutritious and the ones that give you the most in terms of the nutrient to calorie ratio. However, appearances can be deceptive, so stick to the vegetables recommended in the Fat Resistance Diet for the first few months at least.

Unfortunately, most Americans have come to consider corn and potatoes their primary sources of vegetable nourishment. I recently saw a study of U.S. children in which 23 percent of the "vegetables" they ate were in the form of French fries.[6] And the usual American definition of a salad is iceberg lettuce—not great from a nutritional standpoint. Helping you move beyond these bland choices is one of my major goals with the Fat Resistance Diet.

Once you've reeducated your palate, you'll probably have the same experience as most of my patients: you'll find yourself naturally wanting more fruits and vegetables in your diet, choosing instinctively the ones containing the nutrients you need from one day to the next. But you may need a few weeks to adjust to this healthier way of eating. That's why you spend two weeks on Stage 1 and three months on Stage 2 of my Fat Resistance Diet. (See Chapter 6 for more detail.) Still, like Jake, once you get hooked on consuming lots of fruits and veggies, I guarantee you won't want to eat any other way.

So let's replace Myth #1 with Fact #1: *It doesn't matter*

whether a carb is simple or complex. It matters far more what kind of package the carb comes in.

MYTH #2: Carbohydrates can be divided into two categories: low-glycemic and high-glycemic, as measured on the glycemic index. The low-glycemic carbs are good for your health and weight; the high-glycemic carbs are bad.

Again, the truth is more complicated. Yes, there is such a thing as the glycemic index that can be used to measure the glycemic loads of various carbohydrates. A food that potentially inspires a quick upsurge of blood sugar is considered high-glycemic; a food whose effect on blood sugar is slower is considered low-glycemic. But having said this, we haven't really gone very far toward making healthy food choices.

For example, did you know that carrots rate higher on the glycemic index than candy bars? That's because the fat in a candy bar modifies the candy's effect on blood sugar, causing a slower rise. And despite their higher rating on the index, carrots don't give you a quicker blood sugar surge than candy, because carrots are mostly water. So no doctor in the world would advise patients to eat candy bars and avoid carrots. Trust me: I have never seen a patient who gained weight from eating too many carrots.

It's not as though the glycemic index tells us nothing of value. Studies have shown that the more foods you consume that score high on the glycemic index, the more likely you are to have high CRP levels, indicating increased inflammation.[7] But much of the effect noted in these studies was due to foods like white potatoes, low-fiber breakfast cereals, white bread, and white rice—so we're talking about foods that are also low in fiber and other nutrients. In other words, you don't need to know the glycemic index to know that these "white" foods are not a good basis for a healthy diet. So generally, the glycemic index is a pretty rough (and confusing) guide to choosing foods, and I wouldn't advise making it your major focus. Certainly, it wasn't my main consideration in choosing foods for the Fat Resistance Diet. Once again, I've been far more concerned with how rich a food is in fiber and nutrients than in how it performs on the glycemic index. So let's replace Myth #2 with Fact #2: *How a carb performs on the glycemic index matters far less than what kind of package the carb comes in.*

The Right Carbohydrates Help Prevent Diabetes

The worldwide epidemic of type 2 diabetes is associated with an increased risk of heart disease, kidney failure, and stroke. The good news is that our diet has helped readers dramatically improve their health. We have received letters from readers with diabetes who tell us that the Fat Resistance Diet has allowed them lower their blood sugar levels to within the normal range. With these improvements, their doctors have been able to reduce or eliminate the need for medication. These excellent effects are partly due to weight loss and partly due to the beneficial effect of Fat Resistance Foods.

Type 2 diabetes occurs when cells do not respond normally to insulin, a hormone made by the pancreas. This condition is called insulin resistance and leads to high blood sugar, high blood levels of fat (triglycerides), and high blood pressure. A diet based on Fat Resistance Foods helps people with diabetes by reversing insulin resistance. If you don't have diabetes but may be at risk because someone in your family has type 2 diabetes, our diet can help you prevent diabetes by preventing the development of insulin resistance. Here's how it works:

You are more likely to develop insulin resistance if your diet is high in sucrose (table sugar), saturated fat (the kind of fat found in meat and butter), and white starchy foods like white bread, potatoes, and white rice. You are less likely to develop insulin resistance if your diet is high in fiber, omega-3 fats (the kind found in flaxseed and fish), and carotenoids (yellow, orange, and red pigments found in many fruits and vegetables). Several herbs and spices also have antidiabetic effects. The best way to prevent type 2 diabetes is to be physically active and make our meal plans and recipes your diet for life.

In observational studies in different countries, some Fat Resistance Foods have been specifically associated with a reduced risk of developing diabetes. For a few of these, experiments have been done that explain why they can prevent diabetes.

1. Flaxseed. Flaxseed prevents insulin resistance in four ways, making it the king of antidiabetic foods. Flaxseeds are loaded with fiber, omega-3 fats, and carotenoids. They also contain a large amount of lignans, natural compounds shown to reduce insulin resistance in experimental studies. Whole flaxseed is not easily digested, and flaxseed oil lacks the fiber and lignans of whole seeds. The best way to eat flax is to grind organic flaxseed in a coffee grinder every day, to make sure it's fresh. Flaxseeds are easy to find in supermarkets and natural-food stores, and grinding them takes only about 10 seconds. They have a pleasant, nutty flavor. The Fat Resistance Diet gives you many ways to use them.

2. Green tea. Green tea contains natural compounds called flavonoids that reduce inflammation, a leading cause of insulin resistance. Slim Chai Tea, a recipe found in this book, uses spices like cloves, cardamom, and cinnamon to enhance the anti-inflammatory effect of green tea. (More about cinnamon on page 67.)

3. Walnuts and almonds. Walnuts are a source of fiber and omega-3 fats. Almonds contain fiber, essential minerals, and monounsaturated fats. Not only is eating nuts associated with a reduced risk of diabetes, but almonds and walnuts also lower cholesterol in people who already have diabetes.

5. Bell peppers, broccoli, carrots, red cabbage, spinach, and tomatoes. Among the Fat Resistance vegetables, these six are the richest in carotenoids. You'll absorb more carotenoids from these and any other food by cooking them and eating them in a meal that contains some natural sources of fat (like nuts, seeds, salmon or olive oil).

6. Cinnamon. Brewing cinnamon in tea produces an extract that directly increases the sensitivity of your body's cells to insulin. Cinnamon extract also has been shown to reduce the blood sugar of people who already have type 2 diabetes.

7. Garlic, ginger, onion, and turmeric. These tangy spices not only add delicious flavor to the recipes in this book but also combat the inflammation that causes insulin resistance. Each has been shown to reduce blood sugar in scientific experiments.

Fiber and Phytonutrients:
The Key to Choosing Your Carbs

If I didn't rely on the simple/complex dichotomy, and I didn't focus on the glycemic index, what *did* I consider in choosing the carbs to eat on the Fat Resistance Diet? Basically, I looked for foods that were rich in fiber and phytonutrients. Let's take a closer look.

Fiber. Fiber is an indigestible substance with no nutritional value. Yet it is of vital importance to your health and your weight. Fiber is the bulky, fibrous material in fruits and vegetables, nuts and seeds, legumes and whole grains. It passes through your digestive tract without being absorbed. Fiber has a protective effect, because it seems to pick up the toxins and harmful bacteria that accumulate in your digestive tract and move these poisons out through your bowel movements. The consumption of fiber has been associated with a decreased incidence of heart attack and stroke, and a number of studies suggest that it decreases the incidence of colon cancer and gallstones.[8] As you may have noticed, fiber also helps prevent constipation.

You can find fiber in whole grains, nuts, vegetables, and some fruits, including berries. Our ancestors seem to have consumed far more fiber than we do. The federal government recommends 25 grams a day for women and 38 grams a day for men, but the American daily average is only about half that amount. Like many of my medical and scientific colleagues, I think that low fiber consumption contributes to many of our health problems. So in the Fat Resistance Diet, I've chosen fruits and vegetables, nuts and seeds, and eventually legumes and whole grains that will help you increase your fiber consumption. That's because the detoxifying properties of fiber can have a powerful anti-inflammatory effect. A study done at the U.S. government's Centers for Disease Control and Prevention in Atlanta found that the less dietary fiber in a person's diet, the higher the blood CRP levels were likely to be.[9] (As discussed in Chapter 2, CRP levels are a good indicator of inflammation.)

Phytonutrients. *Phyto* means "plant," and *phytonutrients* refers to nutrients found primarily in plants. Phytonutrient is not a scientific term, but it is being used with increasing frequency, and it's one that I find useful to indicate the nutritional value of plants beyond the vitamins and minerals they contain.

Phytonutrients are groups of naturally occurring chemicals found in plant foods that can profoundly influence the function of the cells in your body. They include *carotenoids* and *flavonoids* (also known as *bioflavonoids*).[10] Carotenoids and flavonoids are pigments that give color to food: yellow to deep purple (flavonoids) or pale yellow to bright red (carotenoids).

There are more than four hundred types of flavonoids in the human diet, so I won't try to list them all here, except to point out that berries, cherries, and pomegranates are loaded with them. The best-known carotenoid is beta-carotene, the pigment that makes carrots orange and that helps your body make vitamin A. Tomatoes are a rich source of another carotenoid, lycopene, which helps prevent prostate and ovarian cancer. And the carotenoid lutein, abundant in spinach, helps prevent macular degeneration, a leading cause of blindness.

Here are some other documented health benefits of phytonutrient-rich foods:

- Pomegranate protects against harmful LDL cholesterol.[11]
- Blueberries have been shown to prevent senility in rats— and so, perhaps, in humans as well?[12]

- Tart cherries have been used to treat gout and other types of arthritis.[13]
- Broccoli and other crucifers (cabbage, kale, cauliflower, Brussels sprouts) help prevent breast cancer and other types of cancer.[14]
- Scallions have been shown to protect against prostate cancer.[15]

So here's the formula I've used to choose which carbs you should consume and which you should avoid. I invite you to replace the outdated myths about simple/complex carbs and the glycemic index with this principle:

When choosing carbs, make sure you get the most fiber and phytonutrients in exchange for the calories you consume.

That's it. That's the only principle you really need to remember. And if you follow the Fat Resistance Diet, you won't even need to remember it. You'll be eating that way, every day of your life.

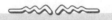

HEALING SPICES

As Jake, the Barbecue King, discovered, herbs and spices have potent anti-inflammatory effects. In addition, these flavorful items contain high levels of minerals and antioxidants, and of course, they enliven the taste of your food. So in preparing the recipes and meal plans for the Fat Resistance Diet, my son Jonathan and I have carefully chosen the herbs and spices that will not only make your meals delicious but will also fight inflammation at the same time.

The centerpiece spices of the Fat Resistance Diet are garlic, onions, scallions, chives, ginger, turmeric, basil, parsley, and cinnamon. Some of these spices have been studied more than others, but all have been shown to have unequivocal health benefits.

(Continued)

Ginger, for example, is a delicious spice that contains some four hundred active components, which perform a wide variety of functions. Ginger can be used to relieve migraine headaches, relieve nausea and morning sickness, and ease the symptoms of arthritis—all testament to ginger's anti-inflammatory properties.[16]

Turmeric contains a group of flavonoids called curcuminoids, which give turmeric its yellow color. Curcuminoids have shown potent anti-inflammatory, anticancer, and detoxifying effects in numerous scientific studies.[17] And cinnamon has recently been shown to increase the response of cells to insulin, improving insulin resistance.[18]

The spices in the Fat Resistance Diet aren't only effective in and of themselves. They also help counteract the inflammatory properties of some animal fats. Whenever you cook any type of animal flesh, including beef and chicken, the cholesterol present in the meat is oxidized and produces a wide variety of damaging substances. Cooked red meat is particularly full of dangerous ingredients known as lipid peroxides, damaged fat molecules that harm tissues and promote inflammation. Interestingly, when red meat is consumed with red wine, ingredients in the wine seem to mitigate the meat's destructive elements—a finding that may indicate a scientific rationale, not just a culinary one, for drinking red wine with meat.[19]

I haven't included red wine in the Fat Resistance Diet, because our recipes for beef actually do an even better job of using spices and condiments to counteract these inflammatory tendencies. We suggest marinating beef in tart cherry concentrate or pomegranate juice, as well as using various combinations of garlic, soy, parsley, rosemary, thyme, pepper, and vegetables in conjunction with the meat.

Fight for Your Right to Eat Well!

As you've probably realized by this point, I didn't start out trying to help my patients lose weight. My focus has always been on supporting patients suffering from inflammation, a condition that is most effectively addressed through nutritional medicine by adding healing foods that have been absent from their diets.

Once I discovered how effective this treatment was as a weight-loss plan, and how different it was from virtually every commercial diet plan on the market, I couldn't help feeling sad. I began to realize how deprived most Americans have been, limited to a few overly sweet tastes and lots of bland, filling, fatty food. The main seasonings we know are salt and ketchup. Our salads are made of iceberg lettuce. Our protein sources are primarily huge portions of barely spiced red meat. And far from educating us into more pleasurable and varied ways of eating, our weight-loss plans are perpetuating the problem. Oh, sure, they might substitute artificial sweeteners for unhealthy white sugar, or offer low-carb or low-fat alternatives to high-calorie food items. But they don't really address the loss of spices, herbs, and fresh produce from the American diet. As a result, we're missing out on one of life's great pleasures: good, fresh, well-seasoned food.

By contrast, traditional cuisines from around the world have long used herbs, spices, and condiments that counteract the inflammatory properties of various foods, especially in combination. As we created the Fat Resistance Diet's recipes and meal plans, my son and I were struck by how traditional Korean cuisine, for example, combines beef or chicken with vegetables and herbs in ways that minimize the harmful properties of lipid peroxides; and how Indian cuisine uses black pepper, which enhances the absorption of flavonoids from turmeric. We took full advantage of this culinary wisdom, marking well how it marries delicious tastes with the healthiest possible food combinations. In offering you the Fat Resistance Diet, we are not only offering you a weight-loss plan. We are also sharing with you our family's passion for delicious, healthy food.

POMEGRANATE

Pomegranates are an excellent example of the healing carbs that make our diet so effective and enjoyable. Pomegranate juice, a star ingredient in many of our recipes, is a convenient way to get the anti-inflammatory benefits of this Fat Resistance food into your day.

People ask me, "Where do I get pomegranate juice?" So here's how to find it: At your local supermarket, check the refrigerated produce section for POM Wonderful unsweetened pomegranate juice. It's got a rich, dark red color and a sweet flavor balanced with a little tartness. Their Web site has a nice feature that helps locate stores that stock the product in the United States and Canada: www.pomwonderful.com.

Summary of Chapter Four:
The Real Truth About Carbs

1. It is a myth that all carbs cause weight gain and should be eliminated.
2. In fact, the right carbs help heal inflammation and promote weight loss.
3. Nutrient-dense carbs contain powerful nutrients that help fight many diseases, including obesity, diabetes, cancer, and arthritis.
4. Choose carbs that are high in fiber and phytonutrients.

five

What's Wrong with Other Diets?

When Emily came to see me for help with losing weight, she was desperate.

"I've been on diets my entire life," she told me. "Either they don't work in the first place, or else they work only for a while. Maybe it's their fault, or maybe it's mine—I know I'm not the most disciplined person in the world."

A fifty-one-year-old executive assistant, Emily had been impressed with the weight-loss results of another woman in her office who had told her that not only had she lost weight with my plan, but she'd also begun to enjoy food in a new way. "Enjoying food sounds good," Emily said wistfully. "I can't remember the last time I put a bite into my mouth without counting calories, carbs, fat grams—whatever."

Emily's attitude did not surprise me. One of the greatest harms that the American obsession with diet has wrought, in my opinion, is the destruction of the pleasure we take in food. Instead of tuning in to our natural hunger and satisfying it with nature's extraordinary palette of tastes, scents, colors, and textures, we've learned to view food in the abstract, in terms of the dangers it poses for our weight and health. Perhaps this wouldn't be so bad if it led us to achieve and maintain a healthy weight, but the fact that the obesity epidemic is getting worse every year is discouraging testimony to the fact that most U.S. diets simply don't work.

Emily's history was a case in point. In her early twenties, she'd tried the original Atkins diet—and gained fifteen pounds. Many people do lose weight, at least temporarily, on a low-carbohydrate, high-protein, high-fat diet of this type, simply because they've cut out refined sugar, white flour, and the harmful trans fats in most baked goods and processed foods—a clear drop in calories that will initially lead to weight loss.

Most people can eat only so much red meat and cheese. Then, they simply stop. But Emily had a voracious appetite for protein, and consuming animal fat and protein in her effort to follow the Atkins plan had loaded her up with saturated fats. So she'd gained weight at an alarming rate and found her cholesterol shooting up as well. Her excessive saturated fat consumption and her weight gain had led to chronic inflammation, with its consequent leptin resistance. From that point on, Emily found it increasingly difficult to keep the pounds off.

In her next attempt at weight loss, she tried the opposite approach—very low fat. Perhaps in reaction to her earlier experience, Emily became a vegan, eating no animal protein in any form—no meat, poultry, fish, dairy products, or eggs. She actually lost thirty-five pounds on this diet during her first year, but mainly because she wound up consuming almost nothing except rice and broccoli.

After three years of living on rice, broccoli, and vitamin/mineral supplements, Emily realized that she was getting sick far too often—a cold or sore throat almost every month. "That was probably the time in my life I was the thinnest," she told me, "but only because I was eating practically nothing and exercising almost all the time. And honestly, I felt terrible. It was my own fault—nothing on the low-fat diet said I had to be quite so narrow in my food choices. But I couldn't make this approach work for me."

Emily decided to get the help of a professional nutritionist, hoping for a more individualized approach that would fit both her personality and her individual biochemistry. The nutritionist seemed helpful at first. She told Emily to eat more protein and to include a greater variety of foods in her diet, based on a system of "food exchanges." Under this approach, Emily was given so many exchanges for dairy, fruit, protein, and so on. In other words, Emily could choose which type of dairy, fruit, or protein she'd eat each day, but she still had to keep count of how many servings of which type of food.

"That was really irritating," Emily reported, although she admitted that at least she stopped getting sick as soon as she reintroduced low-fat, high-protein foods into her diet, including fish, poultry, hard-boiled eggs, and nonfat dairy products. "Except then," Emily continued, "I went into a real weight gain/weight loss yo-yo." First she'd eat more, and she'd gain weight; then she'd cut almost everything out of her diet, and she'd lose weight. "It was getting harder and harder to lose that weight, though," she told me. Psychologically, she grew to hate the crash dieting, and physically, she noticed that each crash diet took off fewer pounds.

In my opinion, Emily had long ago developed chronic low-grade inflammation, aggravated by the yo-yo dieting as well as by her erratic food choices and by the lack of omega-3s and phytonutrients in her diet. But since this perspective wasn't available to her, she continued to flounder. When the Zone diet came out, Emily read the book but decided it was too complicated to follow and even more annoying than the food exchanges. When it became possible to buy all her food prepared according to the Zone from a food service, she tried that for a month, but found that it was too expensive and didn't really satisfy her appetite.

Then *Sugar Busters* was published.[1] Emily bought that book, too, but realized she was already avoiding all the foods the authors said to avoid and she was still struggling with her weight. Clearly, she needed more—but what?

Finally, the South Beach Diet came out. Emily gamely gave it a try, and she did manage to lose a few pounds during the first two weeks—she'd been at the top of her weight cycle when she started. But she never lost any more weight, even after the full twelve weeks on the diet. Her frustration—and her coworker's glowing report—had finally brought her to me.

"Sounds like you hate having to count and quantify everything," I commented when Emily's voice trailed off.

"Yes, exactly!" Emily said, clearly surprised. "I just want someone to tell me what to do."

I thought of how extreme Emily had become when she was following the low-fat diet, and it seemed to me that she needed clear, simple instructions for a very well-balanced eating plan. Whatever diet she was on needed to supply enough variety and flavor to keep her interested and enough inherent balance so that she herself could not unbalance it.

I was in the process of refining the Fat Resistance Diet, so I shared Stages 1 and 2 with Emily and gave her a schedule for eating specific meals at specific times. I knew that such rigidity might help her to have one less thing to think about. And indeed, Emily was delighted to have such explicit directions and even happier to be directed toward meals that were simple, affordable, and yet full of flavor.

For Emily, the Fat Resistance Diet was an unqualified success. She lost ten pounds almost immediately, and gradually continued to lose more. She hasn't gotten sick, doesn't feel imprisoned by the diet, and, best of all, has come to really enjoy what she eats.

Why Other Diets Fail

So what's wrong with America's diet craze? Why do so many of us start out on a diet with good intentions and find ourselves losing a little weight, maybe even a lot of weight—but then within six months or a year, discover we're right back where we started, and maybe even worse off? Why, even if we do keep the weight off, do we feel it's a constant struggle, a battle that never ends, an effort that might easily be sabotaged by a two-week vacation, a few extra desserts, or a busy time at work that interrupts our exercise schedule? And why, in particular, am I seeing so many patients who, like Emily, were unable to achieve long-term weight loss with either Atkins or South Beach?

The reason is very simple: *None of the best-known commercial diets available today provides the nutritional support needed to solve weight-loss problems long-term.*

Either diet might work for you in the short run—after all, millions of people have used both plans for quick weight loss. Even in the short term, however, I've seen numerous patients develop such symptoms as constipation, bloating, fatigue, depression, mental fog, brittle nails, limp hair, and skin problems, not to mention exacerbation of preexisting conditions such as arthritis, asthma, and joint pain. And in the long term, I've known far too many people like Emily, condemned to a lifetime of yo-yo dieting and ever-mounting frustration as their diets work for a while—and then fail.

So in this chapter, I'm going to explain exactly what's wrong with these other popular diets, and why the Fat Resistance Diet avoids their pitfalls. If you've read the first four chapters, you probably already have a pretty good idea of why this plan works and those don't. But I'll say it again: *Other diets don't address the underlying biochemical causes behind weight gain*—inflammation *and the* leptin resistance *it engenders.* True, they may enable a temporary weight loss or even the long-term maintenance of an already healthy weight—but only if you work at it continually. The Fat Resistance Diet is the only eating plan that helps you reverse your biochemical tendency to gain weight and enlists your entire biology on the side of weight loss and weight maintenance, enabling you to lose weight easily and automatically, and keep it off.

Again, if you'd like to skip right to Part Two or Three and get started on the Fat Resistance Diet, that's fine with me. You don't really need to know why other diets don't work to be successful on this one. But if you'd like to understand both the strengths and the weaknesses of Atkins and South Beach, read on. If you've had any experience with either diet, what you read may help you make sense of what happened to you and why you had trouble making those diets work. The problem wasn't your lack of willpower! And if you haven't yet tried them, you can breathe a sigh of relief that you've avoided both the health problems and the yo-yo dieting they can introduce—hazards you won't encounter on the Fat Resistance Diet.

What's Wrong with Atkins—and What's Right with It

Actually, there are two very good things about the Atkins diet:

1. Low-carb diets eliminate some of the major sources of trans fat in the American diet. In Emily's case, cutting out

━━∿∿∿━━

ATKINS'S LOSSES DISAPPEAR AFTER ONLY A YEAR

Research at the University of Washington School of Medicine has found that high-fat, low-carb diets like Atkins actually increase leptin resistance, setting up their participants for a potentially lifelong battle with their appetites and their weight.[2]

Two studies that carefully compared the Atkins plan with other diets found no difference in the amount of weight loss by the time participants had been on the diets for twelve months. In the first study, the Atkins diet was compared to a standard low-fat, low-calorie diet. In the second, conducted at Tufts University, the Atkins diet fared no better than the Ornish regimen, Weight Watchers, or the Zone diet. In fact, the Atkins diet produced the least amount of sustained weight loss of all the diets tested, although the differences were not significant from the perspective of statistical analysis.[3] So while the Atkins approach may seem to provide a quick fix, it won't offer the long-term sustainable weight loss you're looking for. And, as I'll explain further on, it might actually threaten your health.

French fries and carb-containing processed foods meant that she was no longer eating products made with hydrogenated fats. And being allowed to eat butter meant that she was no longer consuming margarine, another major source of trans fats. As we saw in Chapter 3, eliminating trans fats from your diet produces enormous health benefits, including the possible prevention of heart disease and cancer. It also tends to ease inflammation, which in turn leads to a decrease in leptin resistance. So this aspect of low carb is in fact very positive. (Of course, you'll also cut out trans fats and processed foods on the Fat Resistance Diet.)

2. Low-carb diets help you get rid of sugar, white flour, and other empty calories. When Dr. Atkins died, Dean Ornish, whose ultra-low-fat vegetarian plan was the antithesis of the Atkins diet, nevertheless publicly credited Dr. Atkins for alerting the American public to the dangers of sugar. I heartily concur. Any diet that gets Americans to stop eating foods sweetened with processed sugar, corn syrup, and other refined sweeteners can't be all bad. To the extent that the Atkins diet or any other low-carb diet helps people overcome their sugar addiction and their tendency to load up on processed foods, it deserves our applause—and our thanks. (And again, the Fat Resistance Diet will also help you cut out processed sweeteners, white flour, and other empty calories.)

Unfortunately, low-carb diets also pose several problems for dieters:

1. Atkins's theory of carbohydrates is not complete. Dr. Atkins's basic premise is that dietary carbohydrates interfere with fat burning, partly because they encourage your body to produce more insulin, which he sees as a major weight-gain culprit. He's most concerned with two particular effects of insulin: First, it prevents the breakdown of stored fat into fatty acids. Second, it lowers your blood sugar. So if you've eaten a particularly sweet or starchy food, your insulin levels may spike too quickly in response, metabolizing your blood sugar too quickly as well. The result is often a sudden drop in blood sugar, which can leave you feeling dizzy, irritable—and ravenously hungry.

So far, so good. Dr. Atkins is also right to note that in people who suffer from a chronic tendency to low blood sugar (a condition known as *reactive hypoglycemia*), insulin can result in an increased appetite. People who struggle with this condition need to be careful about eating certain types of carbohydrates, especially unaccompanied by protein. Otherwise, consuming the wrong kinds of carbs can provoke the symptoms just noted—dizziness, irritability, and intense hunger.

Hypoglycemia, however, does not necessarily cause obesity. I've had many hypoglycemic patients. Some were obese, to be sure, but most have been thin. It's true that hypoglycemic patients should be careful about eating high-glycemic carbs on an empty stomach—but this in itself is not a major cause of overweight.

While Dr. Atkins puts the blame on insulin itself, in my opinion, it's *insulin resistance* that plays a role in our inability to lose weight. He correctly notes that some obese people—about 25 percent—have high levels of insulin in their blood. And he's right to point out that these high insulin levels work against the breakdown of fat and help to prevent weight loss.

But what's causing these high insulin levels? In Dr. Atkins's view, they're the result of eating too many carbohydrates. Since fat is the only food that doesn't raise insulin levels, his solution is to steer his patients toward a high-fat, low-carb diet, which, he reasons, will keep patients' insulin levels low. Once insulin is no longer sabotaging the body's ability to break down fat and use it for fuel, they can easily lose weight.

Unfortunately, Dr. Atkins was mistaken. Most overweight people don't need to focus on reducing insulin levels. And even if you are among the 25 percent of overweight people suffering from excess insulin, your problem isn't insulin per se, but *insulin resistance*. Let's take a closer look.

Insulin—the hormone your body produces in response to an

increase in blood sugar—has many important benefits. If you're lean and healthy, a sudden increase in insulin after a meal actually suppresses your appetite and stimulates your metabolic rate[4] (exactly the opposite effect from the one Dr. Atkins attributes to it). Insulin has also been shown to help leptin work more effectively, thus enhancing leptin's weight-loss benefits.[5] In other words, when insulin functions normally, it doesn't cause weight gain.

Insulin resistance, however, does. Insulin resistance is a condition found among people—primarily men—whose body fat tends to accumulate around their bellies (as opposed to their hips and thighs), who have high levels of fat (triglycerides) circulating in their blood, and who have a tendency to high blood pressure and diabetes. Together, these symptoms make up a condition known as the *metabolic syndrome*, and for those who suffer from it, it can be deadly.

It's true that people with the metabolic syndrome do better on a diet low in carbs and low on the glycemic index. But you can have the metabolic syndrome and not be overweight—and most overweight people don't suffer from this syndrome. Women, in particular, are less likely to be affected by it, especially if their fat accumulates around their hips and thighs rather than their bellies.

If you *are* among the minority of overweight people who also happen to be insulin-resistant, then you should know that insulin resistance is caused by the same problem that causes leptin resistance: inflammation. In other words, whether you're insulin-resistant or not, you still need to address the underlying problem of inflammation.

Here's where the Atkins diet falls short. Not only won't it cure your inflammation, it will probably make it worse by encouraging you to consume increased amounts of saturated fat (found in red meat, poultry, and dairy products)—a known contributor to inflammation. And if you are insulin-resistant, the Atkins diet will make that problem worse, too: research has shown that your degree of insulin resistance is directly related to the levels of saturated fat in your tissues,[6] levels that are going to be higher if you're eating a lot of red meat and dairy products.

What does this mean in practical terms? It means that if you're among the majority of overweight Americans who are *not* insulin-resistant, reducing insulin levels by restricting all carbohydrates should not be a dietary goal. If you are part of the minority affected by insulin resistance, then yes, you may need to be especially carb conscious at the start of any weight-loss program. Stage 1 of the Fat Resistance Diet will work perfectly for you because it will reduce high insulin levels. *But overcoming insulin resistance does not result from merely lowering insulin levels—it requires the full anti-inflammatory effect of the Fat Resistance Diet, because inflammation is in fact its root cause.*

2. The Atkins diet simply doesn't give you all the elements you need to be truly healthy. Actually, Dr. Atkins was very well aware of this. In his own practice, he prescribed nutritional supplements to make up for the deficiencies in the limited number of foods he allowed you to eat. He wrote books on nutritional supplements and was very familiar with the need for vitamins, minerals, and other nutrients. In theory, if you follow his plan and add a daily regime of pills, you might be able to eke out a healthy routine.

However, we're still learning about all the nutritional components in foods that we need to stay healthy. Science has so far identified only a fraction of the beneficial components in fruits, vegetables, whole grains, and spices. We're just beginning to crack the nutritional code. We may never be able to duplicate nature's bounty in a pill—and we certainly don't know enough to do so now. So to be truly healthy, we should rely as much as possible on fresh, whole foods, and as little as possible on supplementation, recognizing that traditional peoples were quite intelligent about combining foods in ways that bring out their maximum nutritional value.

3. In particular, the Atkins diet doesn't provide nearly enough sources of omega-3 fats. As we saw in Chapter 2, the underlying cause of obesity is not so much insulin resistance as leptin resistance, which in turn is a response to chronic, low-grade inflammation. One of the best things you can do to heal that inflammation and regain your ability to lose weight is to boost your intake of omega-3 fatty acids. Their healing properties to combat inflammation are well known.

But, as we saw in Chapter 3, the more omega-6 fatty acids you're consuming, the more omega-3s you'll need. Besides being overloaded with saturated fat, the Atkins diet has far too many sources of omega-6s—red meat, poultry, and full-fat dairy products—and far too little emphasis on omega-3s, which you get from consuming fish, wild game, and flaxseeds. The imbalance that results sabotages your ability to heal inflammation—and guarantees that your weight will remain high.

4. The Atkins diet poses risks of several side effects. Studies have shown that low-carb diets generally tend to cause fluid loss, which may cause dehydration.[7] Other studies have indicated that a low-carbohydrate diet increases the loss of calcium, which may create an increased risk for osteoporosis,[8] and interferes with the mood-enhancing effects of exercise.[9] Finally, low-carb diets have been associated with increased food cravings—and with bad breath![10]

Where South Beach Goes Right—
and Where It Goes Wrong

At first glance, Dr. Arthur Agatston's South Beach Diet[11] would seem to be a good corrective to the Atkins diet, especially since at least one chapter in the book explaining the diet focuses on why omega-3s are good fats while saturated fats (found in red meat, poultry, and whole-fat dairy products) are bad.

But despite this apparent validation of the importance of omega-3s, the actual South Beach eating plan doesn't do much to promote the consumption of these healthy fats. Unlike the Fat Resistance Diet, which contains several plant and animal sources for omega-3s in all three stages, the South Beach Diet offers relatively few sources for omega-3s—though dieters who've

OTHER LOW-CARB PROS AND CONS

PROS

- *Low-carb diets promote fluid loss.* Low-carb diets do help to lower insulin levels, and one result of lower insulin levels is less fluid retention.
- *Low-carb diets often lead to a quick initial weight loss.* In this way, they can build morale and help people feel that they've regained control over their weight.

CONS

- *Low-carb dieters often suffer from a host of symptoms, including sluggishness, constipation, and poor digestion.* Although they're losing fluid, they're also lacking fiber, which is important for digestive function and a possible hedge against heart disease and cancer.
- *Eventually, you have to add some carbs back into your diet—and low-carb dieters often gain weight as soon as they do.* That's because the low-carb approach conditions you to a high-fat diet, which may help you to feel full. But when you add some carbs, you need to cut back on the fats in order to keep your weight down—and if you've gotten used to a high-fat diet, this can be difficult to do. As a result, many low-carb dieters regain some or all of the weight they lost.

read the book's paean to healthy fats may not be aware of this.

Likewise, South Beach would seem to be on the right track with the notion of "good carbs" and "bad carbs." Rather than avoiding all carbs, Dr. Agatston at least seems to acknowledge that many carbs are beneficial for both health and weight loss.

But again, when you look at how this actually plays out in the diet, you discover that Dr. Agatston has relied entirely on the glycemic index, the scale that tells us what level of blood-sugar increase is produced by consuming a particular food. In his book, high-glycemic carbs are bad; low-glycemic carbs are good. If you want further information about why this is a very problematic way to analyze carbohydrates, look back to page 64 in Chapter 4. Let me just remind you that carrots score higher on the glycemic index than candy bars. So clearly, the glycemic index by itself is not enough to help us make healthy food choices.

Moreover, South Beach is weak in promoting the consumption of phytonutrients and fiber. In Chapter 4 of this book, I discussed why these nutritional elements make some foods Fat Resistance Foods, which both promote weight loss and help us maintain our long-term health. Fat Resistance Foods, I explained, help heal the inflammation that sabotages weight loss, and they're crucial for any short- or long-term dietary plan. You don't identify Fat Resistance Foods by looking at the glycemic index, but by looking at the total package: what vitamins, minerals, phytonutrients, and fiber content a food offers, and what healing powers it has against inflammation and other conditions. The Fat Resistance Diet is based on this concept.

Perhaps the biggest problem with the South Beach Diet is its reliance on artificial sweeteners and fats rather than phytonutrient-rich fruits, seeds, and nuts. Because his diet is focused on reducing insulin, rather than inflammation, Dr. Agatston has ignored the importance of anti-inflammatory carbohydrate-rich foods and either restricted or removed them, using artificial flavoring agents as a replacement. Not only does this undermine the control of inflammation and the reversal of both leptin resistance and insulin resistance, it produces problems of its own. In fact, in addition to the potential dangers of artificial sweeteners, these artificial flavors may actually increase sugar cravings.

American diets have been unnaturally high in overly sweet, oily foods. We've learned that only sweet foods can satisfy our palates and only high-fat items can sate our appetites. The Fat Resistance Diet helps reeducate our bodies and our taste buds, reawakening our appreciation of a wide spectrum of scents and flavors even as it satisfies our hunger with a broad range of healthy foods. South Beach, by contrast, keeps dieters in the same old position of craving sweet and oily foods.

This problem comes out most clearly in South Beach's three phases of dieting. Despite its claim that it is not low carb, Phase One in South Beach is basically a low-fat version of Atkins—a fairly standard low-carb diet. No focus on healing omega-3s; no delicious herbs and spices to retool our palates and ease our inflammation; no profusion of healthy fruits and vegetables to load us up with phytonutrients that will ultimately restore the body's ability to lose and maintain weight.

South Beach's Phase Two is likewise relatively weak from a nutritional standpoint. If you followed every step in South Beach Phase Two, you would fall far short of the nine servings of fruits and vegetables needed each day, and you'd continue to consume artificial sweeteners and fake fats. Moreover, Phase Three is an open invitation to yo-yo dieting. In this maintenance phase of his weight-loss plan, Dr. Agatston suggests that you basically eat what you like. If you gain weight or go off the diet, he says, go back to the more restrictive eating plan of Phase One.

In my view, this is a recipe for disaster. Yo-yo dieting has been shown to impair immune function even as it interferes with weight loss. It may be associated with a slowing of the metabolic rate and it seems to contribute to leptin resistance.

Emily's experience on South Beach illustrates some of the problems. When I analyzed her food consumption, I realized that although she'd been faithfully following the diet, she'd been getting only four or five servings of fruits and vegetables each day—far less than the nine that the National Academy of Sciences (NAS) recommends, and that the Fat Resistance Diet prescribes. As a result, she'd also gotten only about 12 grams of fiber, about half the 25 grams recommended by the NAS, which you will also get on my eating plan.

Moreover, Emily's omega-3 consumption, despite South Beach's ostensible promotion of the importance of these "good fats," never reached the recommended level of 1 percent of her daily calories or 1.5 grams per day, as recommended by the World Health Organization. (Again, you'll get this level of omega-3s on the Fat Resistance Diet.) Emily had grasped the importance of omega-3s from reading the South Beach book, and she tried taking fish oil pills to supplement the diet, but they always made her burp fish oil. Besides, she hated feeling dependent on pills of any kind and was always forgetting to take them. So despite many of the good intentions expressed in the South Beach book, the dietary program really didn't help Emily reshape her food habits, and as a result, her consumption of superfoods—fruits, vegetables, herbs, spices, and rich sources of omega-3s—was pretty low.

The Next Wave

During 2005, there was a surge of public information on the benefits of an anti-inflammatory diet, rich in omega-3s, phytonutrients, and fiber. In his book *Healthy Aging*, Dr. Andrew Weil advocated the benefits of an anti-inflammatory diet for preventing degenerative disease. And Dr. Nicholas Perricone, a dermatologist who had written about the effects of inflammation on aging skin, expanded his work to include an anti-inflammatory weight-loss diet. His professional experience appears to parallel mine in some respects: by giving his patients a diet rich in omega-3 fats and phytonutrients (in his case, to help their skin), he realized that it helped them to lose weight as well. I'm happy to see another physician writing about the connection between obesity and inflammation, as it is vitally important that we help Americans understand the importance of omega-3s, phytonutrients, and fiber. That said, there are a number of important differences between the Fat Resistance Diet and the Perricone program.

The Fat Resistance Diet is specifically designed to heal the primary reason that weight is so hard to lose and so easy to regain: leptin resistance. Dr. Perricone, like Drs. Atkins and Agatston before him, focuses on a secondary feature: insulin and the glycemic index. As a result, his program is essentially a low-carbohydrate diet with a little fruit, barley, buckwheat, and cracked oats added.

These types of diets usually work only in the short run, but long-term they may lead to further weight gain, because they are so hard to maintain and because they don't address leptin resistance—the condition at the very core of weight gain and obesity.

Second, the Fat Resistance Diet does not require nutritional supplements. In contrast, Dr. Perricone's program relies heavily on expensive supplements, which form one of his three steps. But none of the supplements that he recommends has been shown to promote weight loss in people.

Third, the Fat Resistance Diet was carefully designed for your eating pleasure and your convenience. Its Top 40 Super-foods are readily available in your supermarket, and the recipes are custom-made adaptations of classic American and international favorites that are tasty, satisfying, and easy to prepare. I've even made sure to include a daily dessert, because I don't want you to experience a single moment of deprivation or discomfort with this delicious new way of eating. The Perricone program, on the other hand, is built on a number of exotic and hard-to-find foods. Half of his ten "superfoods" are not readily available in many supermarkets.

Furthermore, as a specialist in internal medicine, I designed the Fat Resistance Diet to promote healthy metabolism and good general health, in addition to weight loss. I don't recommend bedtime snacks, because they inhibit the release of growth hormone, an important fat-burning, muscle-building, anti-aging hormone that is primarily released into the bloodstream in the early hours of sleep, reaching a peak at about 1 A.M. It's well known that food eaten too close to bedtime suppresses the release of growth hormone for several hours. However, the Perricone program calls for a substantial bedtime snack every night, not taking into account its suppressive effect on this important metabolic regulator.

The bottom line is that while the Perricone plan is intended to be an anti-inflammatory diet, it doesn't represent the complete picture. The Fat Resistance Diet is tailor-made to address not only insulin resistance but the real key to weight loss: reversing leptin resistance so that your body can start losing weight, and keep it off through its own natural weight-loss mechanism. By focusing on the main problem, leptin resistance, rather than a secondary issue (glycemic index), I have been able to design a diet with a wide range of easily accessible foods and flavors that does not require nutritional supplementation to achieve its anti-inflammatory effects.

The Fat Resistance Diet: A Long-Term Solution

I know that the Fat Resistance Diet works, because I've seen it succeed, time and time again, especially with patients like Emily, for whom virtually every other diet has failed. The Fat Resistance Diet works for a very simple reason: *It's the only diet that's based on the latest scientific understanding of the biochemistry of weight loss.* Of the major commercial diets, the Fat Resistance Diet is the only one to

- heal inflammation and overcome leptin resistance—the major barrier to weight loss
- provide a diet truly rich in omega-3s, phytonutrients, herbs, and spices
- focus on chef-quality meals that are easily prepared with affordable, readily available ingredients
- offer you a lifelong opportunity for weight loss and weight maintenance

I'll let Emily, the lifelong dieter, have the last word. "I never thought I could actually look forward to mealtimes instead of dreading them," she told me the last time I saw her. "Some of that is because this way of eating really does taste good. But some, I know, is because I have finally stopped worrying about doing something wrong. I now know what to eat and what to avoid—and it's such a relief."

WHAT'S IN YOUR DIET?

Diet sodas, low-sugar products, and artificial sweeteners seem to be everywhere, even in other diet books and magazine articles on nutrition. But you won't find any artificial sweeteners in the Fat Resistance Diet, for good reason.

Other diets placate your cravings by "allowing" you sugar substitutes and desserts made with artificial sweeteners. In contrast, our all-natural diet is designed to end your cravings. Readers tell us what a relief it is to have their cravings for sugar and sweets disappear after following our meal plan and recipes. With their cravings gone, they are able to lose weight.

Did you know that artificial sweeteners like those in diet soda can work against weight loss? Studies indicate that they can interfere with your body's ability to regulate intake of calories. This means that you could wind up consuming more calories overall when using artificial sweeteners.

Don't let this news about artificial sweeteners be a best-kept secret. Join the resistance and tell your friends and family. When it comes to our all-natural diet, there is no substitute!

Summary of Chapter Five:
What's Wrong with Other Diets?

1. None of the best-known diets—from Atkins to the Zone—provides the nutritional support needed to solve weight-loss problems long term.
2. Low-fat diets fail to supply the healthy fats necessary for weight loss and well-being.
3. Low-carb diets deprive the body of healing carbs. They can increase inflammation by encouraging you to consume high levels of saturated fat.
4. Only the Fat Resistance Diet treats the root cause of weight gain, which is inflammation and leptin resistance. That's why our plan is so effective in helping readers to lose weight.

PART TWO

The Fat Resistance Diet

six

~~~⌇∿~~~

The Fat Resistance Eating Plan

The Fat Resistance Diet will permanently change the way you think about dieting and about food. You will no longer associate being on a diet with giving something up. Instead, you'll be thinking about the wonderful food you can eat and should eat in order to lose weight. To make this process as easy for you as possible, I've incorporated three steps in designing the menus and recipes:

- All recipes are based on affordable ingredients that you can find easily at any supermarket.
- The recipes require only thirty minutes' preparation time, and most can be made even more quickly than that.
- The recipes were tested and retested, to ensure maximum tastiness and appeal.

In the box at the end of this chapter, I've summarized the guidelines for what you need to eat when dining out on the diet. In the following sections, you can read about the principles I used in creating this weight-loss plan, and learn more about the extraordinary superfoods on which the plan is based.

Each food on the Fat Resistance Diet has been chosen to give you the most flavor, nutritional value, and healing properties for every calorie you consume. I've chosen items that are rich in omega-3 fatty acids, phytonutrients, and fiber, as well as an exquisite array of herbs and spices that will both make your meals taste delicious and help combat inflammation. *Remember, on the Fat Resistance Diet, what you* do *eat is as important as what you don't.* Make sure to consume *all* the different types of foods and spices I recommend to give yourself the greatest possible chance of healing your inflammation, overcoming your leptin resistance, and permanently losing your unwanted weight.

The Twelve Principles of the Fat Resistance Diet

PRINCIPLE #1: CHOOSE FOODS WITH A HIGH NUTRIENT DENSITY

Put simply, this means that you get the most nutritional value for the calories you consume. Every food on the Fat Resistance Diet is rich in one or more of the dietary elements you need to stay healthy, heal your inflammation, and maintain a permanently healthy weight, particularly vitamins, minerals, phytonutrients, fiber, and omega-3 fatty acids. By the same token, you won't see any junk food or empty calories on this eating plan. You won't find any added sugar, artificial sweeteners, or processed fats and oils in any of the recipes.

PRINCIPLE #2: AVOID TRANS FATS

As discussed in Chapter 3, trans fats serve no nutritional purpose and are extremely bad for your health. Trans fats can be found in margarine and in the hydrogenated vegetable oils used in most packaged and processed foods and in most baked goods. Thanks to a new FDA regulation, manufacturers now have to list on every food label how much trans fat is in each serving. There is a pitfall, however, which I explained in Chapter 3. Manufacturers are required to report trans fats only if their level exceeds 0.5 grams per serving. If the labeled serving size is small, a food can still contain significant trans fats. Read labels and avoid foods made with hydrogenated oils, whatever the trans fat content is alleged to be.

PRINCIPLE #3: CONSUME FOODS WITH AN ABUNDANT OMEGA-3 CONTENT

Chapter 3 also showed how omega-3 fatty acids are essential to the healthy functioning of body and brain. Omega-3s help heal inflammation as well as promote a wide range of cellular activities, and they may improve or prevent depression, Alzheimer's disease, cardiac arrhythmias, and a number of other disorders. Plant sources of omega-3s include ground flaxseeds, walnuts, and beans, especially navy, kidney, and soy. Animal sources include fish, especially oily cold-water fish (see Principle #4).

PRINCIPLE #4: EAT FISH AT LEAST THREE TIMES A WEEK

One reason to eat lots of fish is to load on omega-3s. Moreover, studies have shown that eating at least one to two servings of fish per week decreases the risk of sudden cardiac death and of Alzheimer's disease.[1]

What counts as a serving of fish? In research studies, a serving is 3 ounces, about the size of a deck of cards, which should fit in the palm of your hand. And you can even bank the benefits: if you eat an 8-ounce salmon steak, which cooks down to about 6 ounces, you have two servings of fish—not so hard to do.

FLAX: FOR FLAVOR AND HEALING

Flaxseeds (the seeds of the linen plant) are the richest plant food source of alpha-linoleic (ALA) acid, a form of omega-3 fatty acid. In addition to omega-3, flaxseeds are also an excellent source of fiber and phytonutrients, particularly carotenoids and lignans. (Lignans are estrogen-like molecules that may help to prevent the development of breast cancer.)

Ground flaxseeds were the health food of the Romans, incorporated into Roman meal bread. And flaxseed oil has been used as a food oil in central and eastern Europe for centuries.

Because flaxseed oil is unstable, I don't use it in food in the Fat Resistance Diet; this type of oil is best taken as a supplement. But I do use freshly ground flaxseeds in several of my recipes, where you can benefit from their pleasant nutty flavor and crunchy texture.

Although you can buy flaxseed meal, I recommend grinding your own. It's a snap. Buy a coffee grinder that you use only for flaxseeds. Organic flaxseeds are fairly inexpensive, and you can find them at your local supermarket or health food store. Put a tablespoon or two of the flaxseeds in the coffee grinder and grind for about ten seconds. To preserve their freshness and potency and keep the ALA from turning rancid, don't grind the flaxseeds ahead of time; grind them only as needed. (Whole, unground flaxseeds are of little value, because they are so hard they pass intact through your digestive tract.)

PRINCIPLE #5: EAT LOTS OF FIBER— AT LEAST 25 GRAMS PER DAY

Numerous studies have shown that high-fiber diets have an anti-inflammatory effect. For example, a study conducted by the Centers for Disease Control and Prevention found that among nearly 4,000 adults who represented a cross section of

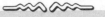

RECOMMENDED FISH

The following fish are both rich in omega-3s and (for the most part) low in mercury, a contaminant found in many freshwater and saltwater fish:

anchovy
conch
herring (fresh or pickled, not creamed)
mackerel, Atlantic only
sablefish
salmon, fresh or smoked
sardines, canned (Atlantic)
sturgeon
tuna, fresh (bluefin, not albacore)

My recipes use primarily salmon and tuna, but any of the fish listed will do.

I also use low-fat (and low-mercury) fish, such as flounder and sole. Although the low fat content of these fish means they're not rich sources of omega-3s, their regular consumption does contribute to your omega-3 intake.

the U.S. population, higher consumption of dietary fiber was correlated with lower levels of CRP, a key indicator of inflammation.[2] In other studies, high fiber intake was associated with protection against heart disease, stroke, and certain kinds of cancer.[3]

High-fiber foods aren't only healthy; they're also bulky and filling. Studies have shown that higher fiber intakes are associated with more satisfaction after a meal and better appetite control, helping to facilitate weight loss.

PRINCIPLE #6: EAT AT LEAST NINE SERVINGS
OF VEGETABLES AND FRUITS EACH DAY

To help you get your nine daily servings, my son Jonathan and I created meal plans and recipes that incorporate fruits and vegetables—particularly those whose deep colors and intense flavors reflect their high content of anti-inflammatory flavonoids and carotenoids—in many delicious ways.

One of the most important groups of phytonutrients is a category known as flavonoids, which give fruits and vegetables their intense flavors and bright colors. Many flavonoids have anti-inflammatory effects that have been demonstrated in scientific studies and are associated with a decreased risk of heart disease and stroke.[4] The human diet potentially includes some four hundred separate flavonoids, but most Americans eat only a tiny fraction of these enticing nutrients.

To get a rough idea of how impoverished most of our diets are, consider this: traditional Asian cuisines supply 4 to 5 grams of flavonoids per day, from tea, spices, herbs, and vegetables; the typical Western diet supplies less than 1 gram per day, mostly from onions and apples.

The deepest red and blue flavonoids belong to a subgroup called anthocyanins, found in the jewel-like colors of fruits such as blueberries, cherries, and pomegranates. I designed the Fat Resistance Diet to include lots of these brilliantly colored foods, making their health benefits available to you every day.

These fruits and their juices are excellent sweeteners, and I use them throughout all stages since they contain such powerful anti-inflammatory flavonoids. Concentrating the fruit juice intensifies the sweetness and concentrates the flavonoids as well.

Another key class of phytonutrients is known as carotenoids, found in carrots, tomatoes, and other yellow, red, and orange foods, as well as spinach. As we saw in Chapter 4, these foods have remarkable healing properties. Carotenoids have antioxidant and anti-inflammatory effects, and their consumption is associated with a decreased risk of cancer and heart disease. The best known is beta-carotene, which helps the body make vitamin A. Lutein, found in spinach, has been shown to protect the retina of the eyes from a condition called macular degeneration, which can lead to blindness. Lycopene, found in tomatoes, decreases the incidence of ovarian cancer and prostate cancer.

It's easier for the body to absorb carotenoids if they're consumed with a little oil or fat.[5] For a large bowl of salad, for example, a teaspoon of oil is needed for maximum absorption. (I recommend olive oil and walnut oil as the healthiest choices.)

Some animal foods contain carotenoids, as well. For example, they're the reason egg yolks are bright yellow, and they help color salmon a deep pink. These foods don't need any additional fat to aid in carotenoid absorption; their natural fat is sufficient.

So what's a serving? For raw vegetables, about a cup; for cooked vegetables, including beans, ½ cup; for fruits and root vegetables, a portion that is about the size of a tennis ball.

PRINCIPLE #7: AVERAGE ONE SERVING DAILY OF ALLIUMS AND CRUCIFERS

- At least four servings per week of allium vegetables (onions, scallions, garlic)
- At least four servings per week of crucifers (broccoli, cauliflower, cabbage, kale, Brussels sprouts)

Both of these classes of vegetables contain special phytonutrients that fight both inflammation and cancer. The cruciferous (cross-bearing) vegetables—known for the cross that you can see within their stems when you slice them open—are particularly important in the prevention of breast cancer. I recommend one serving from each family at least four times a week. Some people don't care for the taste of crucifers, which is actually due to the very chemicals that make them so healthy. I've devised delicious ways of preparing these (try the Sesame Cabbage with

VICTORY THROUGH VEGETABLES

For fighting inflammation, the more colorful your diet, the better. My recipes and menus emphasize those vegetables that are widely available in U.S. markets. I encourage you to eat all the vegetables on this list. There is no restriction on quantity.

arugula

asparagus

bean sprouts

bok choy (Chinese cabbage)

broccoli

Brussels sprouts

cabbage

cauliflower

celery

chives

eggplant

endive

garlic

kale

leeks

lettuce, romaine and red leaf

mushrooms

mustard greens, turnip greens,

collards

okra

onions

parsley

peas

peppers—red, yellow, or green

purslane

radicchio

radishes

scallions

sea vegetables, including

   seaweed

soybeans, sprouted or green

   (edamame)

spinach

squash, summer—zucchini,

   yellow squash

squash, winter—acorn,

   butternut, Hubbard

string beans

Swiss chard

tomatoes

watercress

Carrot, Parsley, and Basil, page 232, or Asian Coleslaw, page 231) that will change your notion of them forever.

A serving of these vegetables is half a cup cooked, one cup raw; a serving of garlic is one small clove.

PRINCIPLE #8: LIMIT SATURATED FAT TO NO MORE THAN 10 PERCENT OF TOTAL CALORIES

- Eat red meat once or twice a week—no more.
- Cook poultry without the skin.

Saturated fat—found in meat and poultry, among other places—promotes inflammation. I provide delicious recipes for enhancing the flavor of skinless poultry. If you season the skin, all the flavor stays on the outside; but in my recipes, the flavor permeates the entire serving.

Cooking red meat generates toxic substances called lipid peroxides and free radicals. But marinating the meat with tart cherry or pomegranate juice both reduces these toxins and enhances the flavor of the meat. When cooking at home for one or two people, an electric grill pan that lets the fat run off is a good way to cook beef.

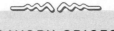

SAVORY SPICES

The herbs and spices listed here have all been shown to contain potent anti-inflammatory compounds—not only in research studies, but among real people eating real food. I use them not only for their anti-inflammatory effects but for the delicious taste they impart to food. I encourage you to use spices of all kinds (except chili, cayenne pepper, and jalapeños), but use these in particular, every day if you can:

basil	cloves
cardamom	ginger
cilantro	parsley
cinnamon	turmeric

PRINCIPLE #9: USE ONLY EGG WHITES OR UNBROKEN EGG YOLKS

Whenever you use eggs, keep the yolk unbroken. If the yolk is broken and then fried or scrambled, the cholesterol in the yolk is oxidized. This produces toxic cholesterol by-products that are far more dangerous than cholesterol itself. A study found that women who consumed fried or scrambled eggs and omelets had an increased risk of ovarian cancer.[6] So poached or hard-boiled whole eggs are fine; otherwise, use egg whites only (they give you high-quality protein and are fat-free). If you think egg whites are boring, check out the recipes for omelets and frittatas—you'll never miss the yolk with all the added vegetables, herbs, and other ingredients, which also give you the phytonutrients.

PRINCIPLE #10: YOU'LL NEVER BE RESTRICTED TO A LOW-FAT DIET

After all, you need fat, both for the anti-inflammatory properties of omega-3 fatty acids and to help you absorb nutrients that dissolve only in fat, such as carotenoids.[7] Throughout, the Fat Resistance Diet provides about 25 to 30 percent of calories from fat.

I do, however, help you keep the healthy ratio of fats that you learned about in Chapter 3 while steering you toward the healthiest possible fat choices. The preferred cooking oils are olive and sesame because they are rich in monounsaturated fats as well as in phytonutrients and antioxidants that keep them from being harmful, even when cooked. The preferred salad oil is walnut, because it tastes wonderful and contains about 10 percent omega-3s. But if you can't find walnut oil or consider it too expensive, use olive oil.

PRINCIPLE #11: EAT TWO HEALTHY SNACKS A DAY

Snacks stave off hunger, and desserts add fun and satisfaction to a meal. Indulge—but in healthy choices only. Using fruits, nuts, and yogurt, I've created delicious snack and dessert treats that will excite your palate while leaving your waistline alone.

PRINCIPLE #12: USE PHYTONUTRIENT-RICH FRUITS FOR SWEETNESS

You don't need refined sugar or artificial sweeteners to create delicious desserts, snacks, marinades, or sauces. Fruits and pure fruit concentrates give you natural sweetness plus anti-inflammatory phytonutrients. The Fat Resistance Diet was designed to make maximum use of sweet superfoods for your eating pleasure. I've emphasized cherry, blueberry, and pomegranate concentrates because they are available year-round and have superior anti-inflammatory effects. Other "natural sweeteners," like brown sugar and honey, cannot compare with these. Brown sugar is basically white sugar with a touch of molasses added back for color and flavor; there is nothing "unrefined" about it. Dark tupelo honey may contain a moderate amount of flavonoids, but most commercially available honey contains little more than sugar.

The Role of Supplements in the Fat Resistance Diet

I've designed the Fat Resistance Diet so that you can get all the nutrients you need from food, not supplements. In fact, I think it's important to get as many crucial nutrients as possible from food, both because it's more fun to eat than to take a vitamin pill and because, truthfully, we don't yet know how many other nutrients or essential elements are contained in the foods we eat.

Nevertheless, people often have special needs that call for higher intake of a particular vitamin or mineral. I've used nutritional supplements extensively in my medical practice, prescribing them to many patients over the years, as well as writing and lecturing about them. In 2004, I received an award

TEA: A SUPER BEVERAGE

Tea is essentially an infusion of vegetable leaves that contain some of the most potent natural anti-inflammatory substances known. Regular consumption of tea, green or black, is associated with a decreased risk of heart disease and the lowered risk of several kinds of cancer, thanks to tea's high content of an ingredient known as catechin polymers. Of these, the most important is epigallocatechin gallate (EGCG); it has potent antioxidant and anti-inflammatory effects, may lower cholesterol in people whose cholesterol is too high, and may also help prevent some kinds of cancer.

You get the most EGCG in young green tea leaves. The older black leaves (which get their color from the fermentation process used) contain more of a flavonoid known as theaflavin, which is also a potent anti-inflammatory substance and a much stronger antioxidant than, for example, vitamin E. Clinical trials of green tea have shown a mild cholesterol-lowering effect and perhaps some benefit for enhancing weight loss.

To enhance the flavor and the anti-inflammatory effects of green tea, I created Slim Chai—green tea with cloves, cardamom, and cinnamon added. If the caffeine bothers you, you can naturally decaffeinate your tea by using the following method:

- Steep the leaves or tea bag in boiling hot water for 60 seconds and discard the water.
- Then steep the leaves again in boiling hot water for 2 to 4 minutes more.

Although most of the caffeine is leached from the leaves in the first minute, it takes 3 to 5 minutes for hot water to fully extract flavonoids from tea.

from the National Nutritional Foods Association—the industry association of health-food stores—for my clinical work in nutritional medicine. I've even designed computer software to help other physicians and health professionals use nutritional supplements properly with patients who are taking medication. So I have a healthy respect for supplements, when properly used.

To address the nutritional requirements described below, I designed a unique multivitamin and mineral formula called Metabolic Cofactors. I originally created it to contain all the vitamins and minerals needed for optimal utilization of omega-3 fats by the body. It's one I take myself every day and use extensively in my medical practice. Metabolic Cofactors is available online at www.fatresistancediet.com.

Nutritional supplementation is very important for the millions of people with special nutritional needs created by:

1. regular use of medication by prescription or over the counter
2. chronic health conditions like diabetes, high blood pressure, digestive problems, or allergies
3. exposure to environmental toxins
4. a stressful lifestyle
5. strenuous exercise
6. genetic factors, suggested by a strong family history of heart disease, cancer, autoimmune disorders, or metabolic problems like osteoporosis or high cholesterol levels

If you do have special needs, my first recommendation is for you to work with a doctor or nutritionist who's skilled in this often controversial area. Some of the supplements most commonly needed by American adults are:

Vitamin D. Vitamin D not only helps you absorb calcium, it also has significant anti-inflammatory, immune-enhancing and anticancer effects.

Low intake of vitamin D is a risk factor for many conditions, including:

- diabetes
- high blood pressure

- heart disease
- cancer (especially colon and prostate)
- autoimmune diseases
- Alzheimer's disease

You need adequate stores of vitamin D in order to lose weight as well. If you're following the Fat Resistance Diet and eating plenty of fish, particularly if you're spending some time each day in the sunlight, you should be getting enough vitamin D. But in northern climates during the winter months, many people become D-deficient. And with the growing use of sun-block to prevent skin cancer, many of us are not absorbing enough D from the sun's rays.

For years in my medical practice, I've been measuring vitamin D levels in the blood of my patients, and a shortage of this crucial vitamin is one of the most common deficiencies I've seen. Scientific research has linked vitamin D deficiency to the development of diabetes, heart disease, osteoporosis, and autoimmune and inflammatory diseases. *Most Americans need 800 to 1,200 units of D_3 a day, taken with a meal.*

A study conducted among women over the age of 55 living in the Midwest found that dietary supplementation with vitamin D_3, at 1,100 IU per day for 4 years, decreased the total cancer incidence by 60 percent. When the researchers confined their analysis to cancer that was diagnosed at least 1 year after supplementation began (a very reasonable adjustment), the decline in cancer incidence reached a whopping 77 percent![8]

Zinc. Low levels of zinc are among the most common nutritional disturbances in the United States. Many Americans attempting to follow healthy diets actually deplete themselves of zinc by choosing foods that are low in this vital mineral. Inflammation further depletes zinc by making it unavailable to your tissues. Zinc is important for detoxification and immunity. Low levels are quite common among people with inflammatory disorders, in part because inflammation actually traps zinc in an unusable form. The Fat Resistance Diet should provide you with an adequate amount of zinc, but if you have recurrent infections, severe allergies, or environmental sensitivities, you may need extra. You may also need supplemental zinc if you:

- take medications to reduce blood pressure, lower stomach acid or control pain or inflammation
- are recovering from surgery
- sweat intensely
- have been exposed to toxic metals like lead or mercury

Zinc supplementation has been shown to be helpful in

- prevention of infection
- treatment of depression
- alleviating attention deficit disorder
- enhancing recovery from inflammatory bowel disease

Atlantic oysters have more zinc than any other food in the world, but they're impractical as a dietary staple or supplement. *You can try a handful of pumpkin seeds every day, or 20 milligrams of zinc in pill form once a day, taken with a meal.* Zinc may be taken as a supplement alone or through a multivitamin/mineral supplement. The ideal zinc supplement would not include calcium and iron, which interfere with the absorption of zinc.

Magnesium. This vital mineral can aid sleep and muscle relaxation. High dietary magnesium helps prevent diabetes, heart disease, osteoporosis, and chronic lung disease. The green vegetables, seafood, and nuts in the Fat Resistance Diet supply ample magnesium, but if you are stressed, exercise intensively, or have environmental sensitivities, you may need more because you're losing so much magnesium each day in sweat or urine. Some symptoms that may indicate a need for extra magnesium include:

- difficulty falling asleep
- muscle tension, cramps, spasms, or twitches

- irritability
- heightened sensitivity to noise
- a "creepy-crawly feeling" under your skin
- palpitations

Magnesium supplements can be very helpful with those symptoms, and the mineral may have some anti-inflammatory effects as well. Magnesium supplementation has been shown to reduce the occurrence of migraine headaches, lower blood pressure, and relieve some symptoms associated with mitral valve prolapse and asthma. Magnesium may cause diarrhea, so you'll have to experiment to find the right dose for you. If your kidneys aren't working properly, you can build up excessive levels of magnesium in your blood, so check with your doctor to make sure your kidneys are healthy. *Then try 100 to 300 milligrams per day, ideally taken at bedtime.* If it doesn't relieve your symptoms within a few weeks, stop taking it and find another way to address those conditions.

Folic Acid. Again, the Fat Resistance Diet is designed to include all the folic acid we need under normal circumstances. But some of us have a genetic defect in how our bodies metabolize this crucial B vitamin. If you're one of those people, you need more folic acid than you'd normally get from a healthy diet.

Here's one way to find out if you need folic acid supplements: Have your doctor give you a blood test for an amino acid known as homocysteine. High blood levels are associated with the common genetic problem I described—and with the need for folic acid supplements. In my opinion, every adult should be tested for homocysteine levels. Because high levels are associated with an increased risk of heart disease, Alzheimer's, osteoporosis, and stroke (as well as having children with birth defects)—and since folic acid supplements reduce homocysteine levels—more and more physicians are routinely screening their patients for elevated homocysteine. If your doctor does find elevated levels of homocysteine in your blood, he or she can recommend a B vitamin or prescribe a preparation that includes folic acid, B_6, and B_{12}.

Calcium. If you follow the Fat Resistance Diet, you should be getting all the calcium you need. But if you're intolerant of dairy or simply don't like it, and if you're not eating the diet's recommended two daily servings of dairy plus lots of greens, then you may need a calcium supplement as well. Try calcium citrate in doses from 500 to 1,000 milligrams, depending on how much calcium (dairy and greens) you're already getting in your diet. *Take 500 milligrams with either one meal or two to boost your intake of this crucial mineral.*

Used properly, calcium can help prevent heartburn and other symptoms associated with hiatal hernia or gastroesophageal reflux disease (GERD). There's been an epidemic of reflux sweeping the country over the past several years, and it follows the epidemic rise of obesity. In fact, being overweight is a significant risk factor for developing GERD. The immediate cause is weakness of the valve that separates the stomach from the esophagus (the LES, or lower esophageal sphincter). Calcium tightens the LES and actually helps your body keep stomach acid out of the esophagus.[9] This is not an antacid effect, because the acidic forms of calcium, like calcium citrate, actually work better than calcium-containing antacids. To be effective, calcium citrate must be taken as a powder so that it dissolves immediately in the stomach. Take one-eighth to one-quarter teaspoon (250 to 500 milligrams) with each meal.

Essential Fatty Acid Supplements

When I was designing the Fat Resistance Diet, I paid special attention to ensuring that you'd get all the essential fatty acids you needed simply by following the guidelines. But some people have special needs for omega-3 and/or omega-6 fatty acids that are hard to achieve through diet alone. Research has shown that fish oil supplements are helpful for people with heart disease, rheumatoid arthritis, psoriasis, asthma, inflammatory bowel disease, dysmenorrhea, and depression, so if you suffer from any of these conditions, you might consider taking supplemental fish oil capsules. Likewise, you might benefit from omega-3 supplementation if by Stage 3 of the Fat Resistance Diet you're still experiencing any of the following symptoms:

- dry or rough skin
- frequent use of moisturizing creams or lotions
- dry or unruly hair
- dandruff
- soft, fraying, or brittle nails
- premenstrual symptoms
- menstrual cramps

I suggest starting with 2,000 milligrams of fish oil each day, making sure you use purified and tested products to avoid the pollutants that might be concentrated in the oils. If you're not getting the results you desire, check with a professional about increasing your dose. Don't raise your dose on your own, however; you might disrupt your digestion or be failing to recognize another cause for your symptoms.

If you're allergic to fish or have other reasons for not consuming fish or fish oils, you can substitute one of three vegetable-derived omega-3 supplements: flaxseed oil, perilla oil, or DHA derived from marine algae. Because the fatty acids in flaxseed oil and perilla oil aren't as potent as those in fish oil, *I recommend a higher dose, about a tablespoon of flaxseed or perilla oil, or a 15,000-milligram capsule per day*. Women should use a flaxseed oil with a high lignan content, which may help prevent the development of breast cancer. Of course, the Fat Resistance Diet, which frequently incorporates ground flaxseed, supplies a generous helping of both essential fatty acids and lignans. *If you're supplementing instead with DHA derived from marine algae, I suggest 250 milligrams per day*.

As for omega-6s, some 85 percent of all Americans get enough of this type of fat from their daily diet and don't need supplementation. However, about 15 percent of all Americans have difficulty processing and using omega-6s, and in that case, it's useful to supplement with a type of omega-6 known as gamma-linolenic acid (GLA), which is not ordinarily consumed in food but has anti-inflammatory effects similar to omega-3s. You can get your GLA quotient in evening primrose, black currant, and borage seed oils. In my experience, GLA is especially useful for women trying to control premenstrual symptoms such as breast pain and swelling or mood swings and for those experiencing perimenopausal sweats and hot flashes. The dose needed is about 300 milligrams per day (or 3,000 milligrams of evening primrose oil). (You can also read more about GLA in my book *Power Healing*, pages 156 to 162.)

Antioxidant Supplements

Antioxidants are important for combating stress caused by inflammation. If you're following the Fat Resistance Diet and eating nine servings of anti-inflammatory fruits and vegetables a day, you shouldn't need antioxidant supplements. Unfortunately, there's been a great deal of confusion in both the popular press and the medical community about antioxidants, so let me try to clear that up.

First, you should know that "antioxidant" is a relative term. Substances that are antioxidant under some circumstances can be pro-oxidant in others. This probably explains why vitamin E and beta-carotene supplements have been getting so much bad press. They're antioxidants (and healthy) under some circumstances, but they function as pro-oxidants (which is unhealthy) in others.

Second, I believe that the vitamins and minerals we've come to praise—including vitamin E, vitamin C, carotenoids, and flavonoids—are really less beneficial because of their antioxidant effects than for other reasons, including their direct anti-inflammatory action. In my opinion, it's far more important to address inflammation than oxidation, even though many of the same vitamins and minerals may be involved.

Third, I'd like to address the matter of the ORAC (oxygen radical absorbance capacity) scale, a device used to measure one aspect of a food's antioxidant capacity. Some health writers are, I believe, misusing this scale. They write as though it's capable of gauging the anti-inflammatory effects of foods—but there's simply no evidence for this claim. You'll find healthy foods at both the high and the low end of the ORAC scale, so it's not a very useful tool for making dietary decisions.

What does this mean in practical terms? Get nine servings of fresh fruits and vegetables each day (which you can easily do by following the Fat Resistance Diet), and don't worry about antioxidant supplements unless you have a medical condition for which they might be needed. You'll lose weight more quickly, improve your health—and save yourself a lot of money!

Green Powders

Green is the color of chlorophyll, found in the leaves and stems of all plants. In most plants, chlorophyll is bound to carotenoids, which protect the plant from stress and damage. Carotenoids are not green. They may be yellow, orange, red or brown. In fruits and roots, where there's little or no chlorophyll, carotenoid colors are visible to the naked eye. Think of carrots (a root vegetable, orange because of beta-carotene) or tomatoes (technically a fruit, red because of lycopene). In the leaves and stems, the carotenoids may be invisible because the intense green of chlorophyll hides their presence. But they're still present. Broccoli, spinach, and parsley are good examples.

Getting enough greens can be difficult, so green drinks are gaining popularity. I spent years investigating the many green drinks and green powders available, looking for one that met my stringent criteria for a truly healthy beverage. Every product failed in one of two important ways:

1. Most green powders are based on grasses (typically wheat grass or barley grass). Grass is a natural food for

grazing animals, like cattle, that have an extra stomach, or rumen, to help digest the tough cell walls of the grasses. Grass is not a normal food for humans and should not be the basis of a health drink.

2. Most green powders contain alfalfa. The sprouts, stems, leaves, and seeds of alfalfa contain a unique amino acid called canavanine, which has been shown to promote autoimmune disease in laboratory experiments.[10] When used as a source of fiber, alfalfa actually produced the opposite effect of other vegetable fibers in an experiment with rats. Typically, vegetable fiber prevents the development of colon cancer in laboratory animals exposed to a cancer-promoting chemical. Feeding alfalfa as a source of fiber actually increased the development of colon cancer in these experiments.[11]

Frustrated by the lack of green powders that were not based on grass or alfalfa, we developed our green powder as an adjunct to the Fat Resistance Diet, based only upon foods that are a normal part of a healthy human diet: carrot, broccoli, cauliflower, spinach, parsley, kale, tomato, blueberry, cherry, cranberry, cinnamon, turmeric, and sea vegetables. We called it SlimGreens because it's a great weight-loss aid. We included sea vegetables (algae) in SlimGreens, because sea vegetables contain a unique carotenoid called fucoxanthin, which studies indicate may help inhibit the growth of fat cells[12] and cancer cells.[13] Use SlimGreens as part of the Fat Resistance Diet in Berry Green Smoothie and Cherry Green Smoothie recipes.

Weight-Loss Supplements

Much of the information I have to impart in this book can start to get pretty complicated, but this part is simple: There is no scientific evidence whatsoever to support the idea that any weight-loss supplement has a significant effect on helping human beings lose weight. Hoodia, chromium picolinate, conjugated linoleic acid (CLA), pyruvate, carnitine—none of these will help you lose weight, so don't waste your money on them, unless there's another reason other than weight loss for you to take them.

There is one exception, however. Green tea concentrate, in a form that supplies 700 milligrams of catechins (a component of the tea), may help you drop a bit of weight. One study found that Japanese men experienced moderate weight loss on that dosage. Green tea contains natural anti-inflammatory substances and may in fact have some weight-loss properties as a result, so it is recommended as a daily beverage in the Fat Resistance Diet.

To order the specific supplements I recommend, including Metabolic Cofactors and SlimGreens, please visit the official Web site of the Fat Resistance Diet, www.fatresistancediet.com.

The Fat Resistance Diet: Weight Loss in Three Stages

I've developed the Fat Resistance Diet with three goals in mind:

- A quick initial weight loss—six to ten pounds within the first two weeks—to boost your morale
- Long-term weight loss at the rate of two pounds per week, to enable you to reach a healthy weight without ever feeling hungry or deprived
- Lifelong maintenance of your healthy weight, which you can achieve effortlessly, having healed your inflammation, overcome your leptin resistance, and reawakened your palate to a whole new range of tastes and flavors

I know that many popular weight-loss plans, including Atkins and South Beach, start with a rapid weight-loss phase in which certain foods are radically restricted. Generally, in these diets, it's dangerous to maintain the initial phase for longer than the time allotted. After that, the body becomes deprived of essential nutrients and severe health problems can result.

That's not the case with the Fat Resistance Diet. If you find it satisfying to remain on Stage 1 indefinitely, feel free. I've designed each of the three stages of this diet to provide you with all the nutrients you need to live a healthy, active life. I personally think it's more interesting to add more varied foods to your diet, as I suggest for Stages 2 and 3, but there is no nutritional reason to be concerned about the length of time you spend on Stage 1.

Likewise, if you are the type of person who resists limiting your diet and wants to start with as many options as possible, go straight to Stage 2 or Stage 3. You won't lose weight nearly as quickly—but you will, eventually, achieve your healthy weight, especially if you follow the suggestions for exercise in Chapter 7. You will also be eating foods that heal your inflammation and help overcome your leptin resistance, enlisting your natural hormonal balance as an ally in your weight-loss and weight-maintenance efforts. If, having begun Stages 2 and 3, you find you want to lose weight more quickly, you can always go on Stage 1 for any length of time you like.

STAGE 1—LOSE SIX TO TEN POUNDS IN TWO WEEKS

This stage of the Fat Resistance Diet is relatively high in protein and low in carbs. That's because when you start to lose weight quickly, you risk losing muscle mass as well as fat. According to Harvard researcher Dr. George Blackburn, you can prevent the loss of muscle with a high protein intake.[14]

Also, studies have shown that people consuming 25 percent to 30 percent of their calories in protein feel more "full" when following weight-reducing diets than people with lower protein intakes.[15] Remember, most Americans consume only about 15 percent of their calories as protein, so to help you feel satisfied during your initial weight-loss stage, I've suggested a higher protein intake.

Finally, Stage 1 is designed to help you quickly lower insulin levels, which may be high in people who are overweight. And, if you happen to be suffering from insulin resistance, the higher-protein, lower-carb approach on Stage 1 will set you on the path to overcoming that condition. (For more on insulin and insulin resistance, see Chapter 5.)

To supply more protein without more saturated fat, I encourage the use of low-fat dairy products as snacks, particularly low-fat cheese (you can now buy some excellent Cheddars that are 75 percent fat-free) and nonfat yogurt. Try your yogurt plain, flavored with fresh or frozen fruit, or sweetened with pure fruit concentrates. But don't buy commercial flavored yogurt of any type—it's loaded with sugar.

STAGE 2—LOSE TWO POUNDS PER WEEK UNTIL YOU ACHIEVE YOUR IDEAL WEIGHT

This is the heart of the Fat Resistance Diet, intended to help you achieve persistent weight loss until you reach your ideal weight. Basically, you continue the eating habits you established in Stage 1, but you add some grains and legumes (beans, chickpeas, lentils) to include relatively more carbohydrates, along with quite a bit more fiber.

The initial weight loss in Stage 1, along with the decrease in inflammation and the improvement in your nutritional status, means that if you are one of the minority for whom insulin levels are a concern, you no longer have to focus on them. In any case, the worst offenders among high-glycemic foods (i.e., those most likely to make your insulin levels spike) are not included in any stage of the Fat Resistance Diet. And because your weight loss will be more sustained and less dramatic, you don't need to concentrate quite so much on ensuring a high protein intake.

Besides the variety that grains and legumes add to your diet, the extra fiber they contribute is good for your overall health. Adding

DINING OUT ON THE FAT RESISTANCE DIET, STAGE I

BREAKFAST CHOICES

1. Egg white omelets and frittatas with smoked salmon or 1 ounce of low-fat cheese; tomatoes, spinach, or other vegetables.
2. Eight ounces of nonfat plain yogurt with a few walnuts or almonds and a serving of fresh fruit.
3. Smoothie with nonfat plain yogurt, whey or soy protein, and fresh fruit.
4. Two hard-boiled eggs with tomato or other vegetables and half a grapefruit.

LUNCH CHOICES

1. Wraps, made with three large leaves of fresh romaine lettuce instead of bread; 6 ounces of roast chicken, roast turkey, tuna, or salmon; and vegetables, such as tomatoes, onions, scallions, or shredded carrots.
2. Salads with fresh dark greens and a variety of vegetables and fruits: tomatoes, carrots, string beans, broccoli florets; apple, orange, or grapefruit slices; 1 teaspoon of olive oil; vinegar or lemon juice; and *one* of the following:

   - 1 hard-boiled egg
   - 2 ounces of low-fat cheese or a cup of low-fat cottage cheese
   - 6 ounces of tuna or salmon

SUPPLEMENT YOUR SANDWICH OR A SALAD WITH SOUP

Eat vegetable soups made without cream, oil, flour, potatoes, corn, or sugar—just vegetables, spices, water, and broth.

DINNER CHOICES

1. Fish, three or more times a week, boiled or baked without added fat. Order as many grilled or roasted vegetables (except corn or potatoes) as you like.
2. Chicken or turkey, up to four times a week, broiled or roasted without the skin, flavored with herbs and spices. I recommend a serving

(Continued)

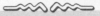

size of 4 to 8 ounces. Order with as many types of grilled or roasted vegetables (except corn or potatoes) as you like.

3. Beef; no more than once a week. Order lean cuts like sirloin or flank steak, and limit portion size to 6 ounces (two decks of cards) or less. No sauces except marinades. Order with lots of vegetables (except corn or potatoes).

4. Vegetarian dinners, at least once a week. Order steamed vegetables (except corn or potatoes), with tofu or tempeh for added protein (no limit on vegetable portions; keep tofu or tempeh below 8 ounces). Add soy sauce for flavor.

DESSERTS

Choose one dessert each day:

1. A serving of fresh fruit.
2. A cup of nonfat plain yogurt with a serving of fruit, such as berries.

BEVERAGES

1. Green or black tea.
2. Vegetable and fruit juices.
3. Spritzers made from seltzer or sparkling mineral water and fruit juice, one to two glasses a day.
4. Coffee: preferably decaffeinated, no more than one cup a day.
5. Low-fat milk or unsweetened soymilk, no more than two glasses a day.

grains and legumes also makes it possible to suggest more vegetarian meals, helping you keep your vegetable consumption high.

In Stage 2 you'll also find the addition of some fruits with more sweetness and a higher glycemic index, like pineapple and figs. Having rebalanced your insulin levels in Stage 1, your body will have an easier time handling the glycemic effect of these fruits. And, again, they make eating more fun!

ON THE RUN: 100-CALORIE DIET-SAVER SNACKS

DAIRY

¾ cup (6 ounces) of nonfat plain yogurt; or add

1 teaspoon of unsweetened blueberry or tart cherry concentrate or

2 tablespoons pomegranate juice to

½ cup (4 ounces) of nonfat plain yogurt

½ cup (4 ounces) of low-fat cottage cheese

1 ounce of low-fat hard cheese (Cheddar, Monterey Jack)

1 low-fat mozzarella stick

1 cup of nonfat or 1 percent milk

1 scoop of whey protein concentrate in water

FRUIT

1 large apple

1 large pear

1 cup of fresh or frozen blueberries

1 cup of fresh cherries

1 large nectarine

2 medium peaches

2 cups of grapes

2 kiwis

1 large orange

1 medium grapefruit

½ cup of unsweetened applesauce

JUICE

9 ounces of grapefruit juice

8 ounces of vegetable juice

Spritzers made from sparkling mineral water and the juice of a lime or lemon or 1 teaspoon of unsweetened blueberry or tart cherry concentrate or 2 tablespoons of pomegranate juice

(Continued)

NUTS AND SEEDS (RAW OR DRY-ROASTED)

12 raw almonds

8 walnut halves

4 Brazil nuts

¾ ounce of pumpkin seeds

VEGETABLES

1 cup of fresh, crunchy vegetables: celery, carrots, broccoli, or cauliflower. These can be dipped in almond butter (up to 1 teaspoon), if desired.

2 scoops of SlimGreens in water with 1 teaspoon of unsweetened blueberry or tart cherry concentrate or 2 tablespoons of pomegranate juice (see Resources). Visit www.fatresistancediet.com for SlimGreens.

STAGE 3—MAINTAIN YOUR IDEAL WEIGHT

Once you've achieved your ideal weight and your body responds to food in a normal fashion, you can start eating potatoes, pasta, and a wide variety of whole-grain foods—including whole wheat bread. Continue to avoid deep-fried foods, though, and foods made with refined sugar or unhealthy fats. By this point, your own instincts will lead you to the healthiest possible food choices. By the time you reach Stage 3, you will have become your own diet doctor, but we still get you started in this final stage with two weeks of menus and more amazing recipes.

The important thing for all three stages is to begin taking pleasure in every bite you eat—a goal that is just as important to me as helping you lose weight or heal your inflammation. Understand that if you don't enjoy what you're eating, you won't stay on this diet for long. Pleasure in eating and drinking can be one of your most important allies in achieving and maintaining the body you hope for. That's why we've created recipes that maximize enjoyment as well as nutrition. Sharing the joy of healthy, delicious foods is a key part of the Fat Resistance Diet.

Flexible and Fun Tips for Fat Resistance

We designed the Fat Resistance Diet to be flexible and fun.

Sometimes readers wonder if the diet is effective in cases where they can't eat a particular food. The Fat Resistance Diet does not rely upon a particular ingredient but instead is based on maximizing nutrition and eating pleasure. If you cannot eat a particular ingredient because of an allergy or another reason, you'll find many delicious alternatives suggested throughout the book. Our family follows the principles in a flexible way, with healthy and delicious meals and snacks. You can, too!

The meal plans in our book were carefully created to produce the fastest weight loss. But you can join the Fat Resistance lifestyle one meal at a time in any way that works for you. If your preference is for dairy-free recipes, we have lots of those. Are you looking for vegan recipes? You have come to the right place because this book is loaded with recipes that are vegan-friendly. Here are some practical tips to help you get started.

First, identify your greatest food challenge: Is it finding time to eat a nutritious and satisfying breakfast, dealing with the day-time munchies, craving an after-dinner sweet, drinking too many calories or too much sugar, always wanting a second helping, or eating out frequently? You can use the Fat Resistance Diet to handle these challenges.

If breakfast is the challenge, find a breakfast recipe in our book that appeals to you and have it every morning, if you like. The Smart Start Smoothie can be made quickly and packs enough anti-inflammatory nutrition to get you through the morning.

If the munchies are your challenge: Take a look at the

"100-Calorie Diet Savers" in Chapter Six, choose the ones with most appeal, and keep them handy. Grab a handful of walnuts, and you get healthy omega fats. Or use any of the morning or afternoon snacks in Stage 1 or 2. One of our favorite snacks is to add a tablespoon of SlimGreens to a cup of vegetable juice. For SlimGreens, go to www.fatresistancediet.com.

If desserts do you in, check out the nutritious, delicious desserts in Stages 1 and 2, select the ones you like best, and eat one every night. Even our amazing Black Forest Banana Split will not interfere with weight loss.

Are soft drinks or fruit juices or cappuccino your undoing? Then try these beverage ideas: Our Iced Mocha Latte is a delicious and satisfying drink. Spices give our Slim Chai Tea an aroma and flavor you'll love. If you like your drinks cold and bubbly, make Pomegranate Spritzers. Keep a supply of sparkling mineral water on hand, and add ice and pomegranate juice to your desired level of sweetness.

If you generally favor large portions or second helpings, try starting your meal with one of our soups. Immune Power Soup is a great favorite of our family and friends. Make a large batch once a week, divide it into portions, and freeze them. Thaw and heat one portion a day.

If you eat out frequently and prepare few of your own meals, the suggestions for "Dining Out on the Fat Resistance Diet" in Chapter Six will help you choose your meals wisely.

As an example of the recipes you can enjoy if you have a food preference, here's a list of our vegan-friendly recipes, for those looking for recipes made without animal-derived ingredients.

STAGE 1 VEGAN-FRIENDLY RECIPES

Crispy Tofu
Gazpacho

Mexican Salad
Grilled Vegetables with Tofu
Big Vegetable Bowl
Slim Chai Tea
Iced Mocha Latte
Pomegranate Lime Dressing
Immune Power Soup
Garden Salad
Pesto Vinaigrette
Asparagus with Red Bell Pepper and Garlic
Asian Coleslaw
Sesame Cabbage with Carrot, Parsley, and Basil
Cinnamon Lemon Poached Pears with Cherry Syrup
Fruit Kebabs with Pomegranate Glaze
Baked Apples with Cinnamon and Walnuts
Strawberry-Mango Granita

STAGE 2 VEGAN-FRIENDLY RECIPES

Omega Blast Granola
Blueberry Cinnamon Bowl
Basmati Rice Salad
Winter Warm Tomato Basil Soup
Insalata Fagioli
Herb Hummus Wrap
Fifteen-Minute Chili
Ginger Orange Dressing
Zucchini with Garlic and Herbs
Lemon Spice Dressing
Vine-Ripened Tomato Salad
Pineapple Orange Granita
Warm Spiced Apricots and Figs
Fried Bananas

STAGE 3 VEGAN-FRIENDLY RECIPES

Hummus and Greens on Tortilla
Pasta with Tuscan White Beans
Minestrone Rustica
Vegetarian Curry
Spinach Leek Soup

Those who prefer dairy-free recipes will find many choices on our diet. Going dairy-free is made easier because none of the recipes use butter or cream. As a first step, check the ingredient list and choose recipes without nonfat milk, nonfat yogurt, or cheese of any type. Next, if you prefer using soy products, try substituting soymilk or soy yogurt. For example, we made the Blueberry Flax Pancakes in Stage 3 using soymilk, and they turned out great!

Remember that the Fat Resistance Diet is more than a diet. It's really a way of thinking about food with the purpose of helping all of us move toward a healthier lifestyle.

Summary of Chapter Six:
The Fat Resistance Eating Plan

1. Nutritional medicine provides the scientific basis for what the body needs to lose weight and maintain health.
2. Twelve principles for optimizing nutrition guide The Fat Resistance Diet.
3. The meal plan and recipes put it all together into an effective program.
4. Our diet is a revelation for many of our readers, who are delighted to find out how delicious and satisfying healthy eating can be.

seven

〜〜〜

The Joy of Movement:
How Exercise Can Help You
Overcome Leptin Resistance

don't know what to do about this, Doctor. I'm at my wit's end."

Ruby was a thirty-five-year-old social worker, married and the mother of a five-year-old child. She'd struggled with a weight problem most of her life. As an adult, she'd followed a rigidly disciplined diet and exercise plan: 1,500 to 1,800 calories per day, low in fat and sugar, high in vegetables and fiber; supported by a one-hour gym workout three days a week, generally using the elliptical machine, the StairMaster, and various resistance machines.

"But then I'm always injuring myself," Ruby explained. "And then I can't exercise. And then I gain weight."

Ruby went on to detail the pattern that had prevailed for the past few years. She'd start out at the gym, full of good intentions. One day, she'd awaken with a severe pain in her knee, back, or shoulder—pain so intense that she had to move gingerly throughout the day and couldn't even consider returning for her next workout. Discouraged, she'd eat more to console herself, and her weight would rise. Eventually, she'd snap out of it, return to the gym and to her restricted diet, and she'd lose the pounds she'd put on. And then, within a few weeks or a few months, she'd injure herself, and the cycle would start all over again.

When I shared with her the Fat Resistance Diet, her eyes lit up. "You mean I can eat all this and still not gain weight?" she asked me. I assured her it was true. Ruby was sufficiently disciplined and had a good enough understanding of nutrition that she immediately felt confident about implementing my eating plan, and she could see right away that it would be easy to follow.

But we both knew that if Ruby continued to injure herself, she would have a difficult time stabilizing her weight. Not only did she need the weight-loss benefits of moving vigorously and burning off a certain number of calories; she also needed the anti-inflammatory protection that exercise seems to provide. As I've said throughout this book, inflammation is a complicated process that is affected by a number of different elements, including dietary choices, obesity, stress, and exposure to environmental and food-based toxins. (We'll explore the latter two elements in Chapters 8 and 9.) I explained to Ruby that regular, moderate exercise has enormous anti-inflammatory benefits that could help her defeat her leptin resistance once and for all, ensuring that she would remain at a healthy weight.

"But I *can't* exercise if I'm injured, can I?" she asked. "I'll only hurt myself more."

That was perfectly true, I agreed. But there was a reason she was prone to so many injuries: her exercise program had ignored the fundamentals.

Ruby's lifelong commitment to exercise had left her with a good aerobic capacity and a fair amount of strength and endurance in her arms and legs. Yet her devotion to gym workouts and muscle toning had led her to ignore the strength, stability, and flexibility of the muscles that stabilize pivotal points in the core of her body: the muscles of her pelvic floor, the back of her thighs, her shoulders, and the transverse abdominal muscles.

The StairMaster, for example, works the quadriceps in front of the thighs—but totally neglects the hamstrings at the back of the thighs. In Ruby's case, this discrepancy between front and back made her knees susceptible to injury. Moreover, her pregnancy had weakened the muscles of the pelvic floor. And while Ruby told me proudly that she could do up to three hundred sit-ups, she didn't realize that sit-ups don't strengthen the muscles that are essential for flattening the abdomen and stabilizing the spine, preventing injury. As a result of all these imbalances, Ruby was susceptible to knee, back, and shoulder injuries—and that's exactly what she'd been getting.

"But I do lots of stretches," Ruby protested, when I explained my concerns.

"Let me guess," I replied. "Most of your stretches involve touching your toes while you're standing—am I right?"

She looked at me in surprise. "How did you know?"

I explained that standing stretches of the kind she was used to actually stretched the spinal ligaments instead of the hamstring muscles. Combined with a weak pelvic floor and lax ligaments in the back, Ruby's tight hamstrings had left her extremely susceptible to back pain. Her neglect of her transverse abdominal muscles only worsened the problem.

"Try my exercise program for a few weeks," I suggested. But when I explained my basic routine for strengthening, stabilizing, and stretching the core muscles—a routine that works equally well for veteran exercisers like Ruby and for deconditioned people who need to start slowly—Ruby balked.

"These look way too simple," she told me. "They seem like exercises for beginners."

"When it comes to preventing injury, you are a beginner," I told her. "In my experience, even competitive athletes can benefit from this program. If you're very fit or very strong, you can make some simple modifications that will make this routine more challenging. But unless you're a trained dancer or gymnast, you're going to see benefits from this approach. Just try it."

Ruby agreed to give my approach a try. And indeed, after only a few days, she began to feel the difference.

"It's subtle, but it's definitely there," she told me the next time we met. "I feel stronger in ways I've never felt before—almost like I'm 'knit together' more securely. And so far—no injuries!" Three years later, Ruby was still injury-free. And the combination of the Fat Resistance Diet and regular exercise has made maintaining a healthy weight seem effortless indeed.

Exercise for Health, Weight Loss—and Pleasure!

Just as our culture has turned the pleasures of eating into a choice between sweet, oily foods and restrictive diets, so have we transformed the joy of movement into "exercise," a regimented form of activity that many of us resist. Our lives are set up so that we move as little as possible—sedentary jobs that can't be reached on foot or by bicycle; activities that require driving our kids long distances; suburbs and small towns set up to discourage pedestrian and bike traffic.

So let me start by giving you the good news: *Even a slight increase in physical activity can benefit your health.* And if you're one of those Americans who, according to national statistics, gets very little exercise, the news is even better for you, because just about any kind of movement you add into your life will help you get healthy, lose weight, and rediscover the joy of movement.

In a moment, I'll go through the scientific benefits of exercise—how movement helps combat inflammation, overcome leptin resistance, and support a lifelong ability to maintain your weight, as you continue to follow the Fat Resistance Diet. But first, just as I want you to reconnect to the pleasures of eating a wide variety of flavors and textures, I also want to help you regain the joy of moving and using your body.

Think for a moment of children who have just learned to walk, or toddlers who are still amazed that they can propel themselves through space. They move not to lose weight or to strengthen their hearts, but simply for the joy of moving. On some level, they understand that their bodies are *designed* for movement.

Significantly, most healthy toddlers are in such terrific physical shape for their size that they'd put even the most accomplished adult athlete to shame. A famous study was once done in which professional football players were paired with toddlers and asked to imitate every single one of the toddlers' movements. To everyone's surprise, the toddlers had more stamina than the athletes!

I'm not expecting you to equal the strength and endurance of a pro ballplayer—or even of a two-year-old child. But I am hoping you'll reconnect to your body through movement and mild exertion. If you haven't been active in a while, by all means, *start slowly*. Take a walk around the block, pull some weeds out of your garden, or even push a vacuum cleaner around your home. Just about anything you do that involves physical movement—even standing rather than sitting as you return a phone call or chop onions for dinner—burns some calories and helps you lose weight. More important, it starts reconnecting you to the physical pleasure of using your body.

Exercise and Inflammation

There are lots of ways in which exercise can help you lose weight (see the box "Little by Little" on page 143). But one of the most significant is also one of the least known. People who engage in regular, moderate physical exercise experience a

HOW MOVING HELPS YOU LOSE WEIGHT

• **Moving burns calories.** Even activities that aren't strenuous, such as walking at a modest pace, burn up 70 percent more calories per minute than just sitting and watching television. The more time you spend moving, or at least standing, the more calories you burn—and the easier it is to lose and maintain weight loss. The National Weight Control Registry keeps track of thousands of people who overcame dangerous levels of obesity and have maintained their weight loss for at least five years. *The one thing they all share is an increased level of physical activity.*[1]

• **Moving tones and strengthens muscles.** The more muscle you have, the faster your metabolic rate, and the easier it is to lose weight. By the same token, the less muscle you have, the lower your metabolic rate and the harder it is to lose weight.

• **Moving combats aging.** If you develop the habit of moving regularly, even if you're already forty, fifty, sixty, or older, you'll start to combat the effects of aging. On a practical level, strong, well-toned muscles help protect your joints and ligaments from injury—another hazard frequently associated with old age. Besides, toned muscles just look better!

• **Moving improves immunity and mood.** Numerous studies have shown that even moderate physical activity helps people ward off colds and overcome depression.[2] In fact, when it comes to your mood and immune system, moderate activity is just as good as or, in some cases, even better than strenuous activity. A more upbeat mood helps you avoid the stress-induced eating that makes so many people add pounds. And a strong immune system wards off the common viral infections that can be a source of fatigue and keep you from enjoying physical movement.

significant anti-inflammatory effect, as indicated by the lower blood levels of C-reactive protein (CRP). (As you'll recall from Chapter 2, CRP is a key indicator of inflammation that may also help cause it.)[3] Moreover, a recent study of adult men found that those who engaged in three hours a week of moderate aerobic activity showed an increase in leptin sensitivity, suggesting that exercise directly combats leptin resistance.[4]

We don't yet know exactly how exercise works on inflammation or leptin. But we do know that *regular* exercise is the key. Being a weekend warrior isn't nearly as effective against inflammation as getting in some moderate activity most days of the week.

The World Health Organization (WHO) currently recommends an hour a day of moderate-intensity physical activity on most days of the week, for maintaining a healthy body weight and preventing chronic disease.[5] Moderate-intensity exercise includes brisk walking (about three miles an hour), gardening, vigorous housework, dancing, yoga, t'ai chi, cycling, or swimming. If, like most of us, your lifestyle is sedentary, the WHO guidelines are an excellent goal and not hard to achieve. The hour of activity does not have to be continuous. You do not need to spend an hour a day at the gym to get the job done. Think in ten-minute segments. A brisk ten-minute walk from the far end of the parking lot to your office, plus the same ten-minute walk back to your car, gets you a third of the way there. If you add twenty minutes on a stationary bicycle while watching the news and another twenty minutes cleaning your home, you've met the WHO goal for your day. If you enjoy more strenuous forms of activity, by all means pursue them. Some fitness experts advocate weight lifting for weight loss and body toning. Although working out with weights can build muscle, it has less effect on combating inflammation and leptin resistance than regular aerobic exercise. Aerobic exercise involves continuous muscle activity that lasts for at least ninety seconds, rhythmically working large muscles, like those in your legs, and increasing your body's consumption of oxygen. Walking, dancing, and t'ai chi do this much better than lifting weights.

It's interesting to compare the WHO recommendations with the work of anthropologist S. Boyd Eaton. Eaton argues that the

YOUR BASIC ANTI-INFLAMMATORY MOVEMENT PLAN

As I've said, I want you to start slow. You're much more likely to enjoy movement if the pace is right for you! Here is the healthy minimum level of movement that you should try to achieve eventually for optimum weight-loss and anti-inflammatory effect.

- Five hours a week: walking, housekeeping, gardening, yoga, t'ai chi, or some other form of moderate aerobic activity. Do these activities no fewer than five days a week, for a total of five hours:

    5 days/week = 1 hour/day
    6 days/week = 50 minutes/day
    7 days/week = 45 minutes/day

- Core-strengthening exercises at least three times a week. (See page 135.) If you're already engaging in strength training or resistance training, follow my core exercise plan before every workout.

human genome—our genetic heritage—is out of sync with our modern lifestyle and best suited to the lifestyles of Stone Age humans, who gathered food and stalked wild game for tens of thousands of years. Our ancestors spent much of their time looking for food, but they were not endurance athletes. They also spent much of their time sleeping, socializing, relaxing, and creating language, myth, and culture. Eaton estimates that the average Stone Age adult burned about 500 calories a day through physical activity of moderate intensity, an amount of exercise that is quite consistent with the WHO guidelines.[6] By following the guidelines, we can match modern lifestyles with ancient genes, improve our health and energy, and manage our weight.

Walking: Your Easiest Weight-Loss Aid

Walking is wonderful exercise, involving the entire body—and, if you walk with awareness and appreciation of your surroundings, it can involve your mind and spirit as well. Walking beside the ocean, through the woods, or along a fascinating city street is a pleasure for its own sake, in addition to the health and weight-loss benefits that it brings. Even walking briskly through a mall—a suburban alternative—can be a pleasure, as your breathing deepens, your mind quickens, and your body starts to come alive.

Please look for opportunities to build more walking into your daily routine. Just begin moving, even a little at a time. The more you move, the more you want to move—and the more weight you lose, enabling you to move more easily and enjoyably. Your muscles and lungs grow stronger, your heart and circulation work more efficiently, and sooner or later, you're eager for movement, hungry for it, as one of your most cherished pleasures. You're also healing your inflammation, slowly but surely, with every step you take.

Walk briskly from the far end of the parking lot to your office door; climb the stairs rather than taking the elevator. Get off one stop early if you take the bus or subway, and walk the rest of the way. Park as far as you safely can from where you're going and build in an extra stroll. Add a ten-minute walk to your lunch hour. Before you do your grocery shopping, take a brisk walk up and down the aisles, scanning quickly for specials and items you'd forgotten that you needed. Or walk around the whole shopping mall before going in a store.

In other words, look for opportunities to walk as much as possible throughout the day, knowing that each step you take adds up to more muscle tone, more weight lost, and more inflammation healed. Make it a game—where can you add a few extra steps? Start small—but start somewhere.

One of the great things about walking is that you don't need any equipment except a comfortable pair of shoes. But make sure that your shoes *are* comfortable, and that they have some relationship to the shape of your foot. A good walking shoe should be wide in the toes and widest across the ball of the foot. It should be snug at the heel, so there's no slippage, and well supported in the arch. If your feet hurt when walking, consider trying a different shoe.

The average sedentary American woman takes fewer than 6,000 steps a day. And studies have shown that people who walk fewer than 5,000 steps per day are more likely to be overweight, while those who walk more than 9,000 steps per day are more likely to be of normal weight.[7] In fact, the number of steps you take each day is directly associated with the size of your waist and hips.[8] So your goal should be to add about 5,000 steps, which you can easily do by taking a moderately paced thirty- or forty-minute walk. If that sounds like too much right now, start with a five-minute daily walk, and every week, add five more minutes. You may find yourself looking forward to that brief time of movement as the high point of your day!

ARE YOU EXERCISING TOO HARD?

Here's a basic rule of thumb: *Moderate activity is invigorating. Strenuous activity causes fatigue.* If movement doesn't leave you feeling better, then it was too intense for your fitness level. While moderate exercise helps combat inflammation, excessive exercise can actively increase the inflammation it was meant to heal.[9] So if you end a session feeling fatigued or out of sorts, don't give up; just back down and build up more slowly.

Strengthening Your Core

The most important muscles are those you don't see. They stabilize your torso, improve your posture, and make you more flexible. If you want to avoid injury, you need to take care of these muscles—and they'll also help you to stand tall and look trim. Here's a series of six activities that will help you strengthen your core. They take about fifteen minutes in all, and they're well worth the effort. Even if you can't do the whole cycle of six, try to spend at least two to three minutes each morning doing the first one. (I've also included one knee strengthener, which will help prevent injury and keep you limber.)

1. SERENITY CROUCH

WARM-UP:
- Stand in a comfortable position with your feet a bit more than shoulder width apart.
- Bend your knees slightly to lower your buttocks about an inch or two. (This is a very mild squat; it should cause no discomfort at all.)
- Swing your arms loosely and lightly from front to back and back to front, so that each arm comes forward as the other arm swings back. Let your knees bend and straighten with the rhythm of your arms, causing your torso to bob up and down gently. Continue for about half a minute.

THE EXERCISE:
- Hold this relaxed squat—your feet spaced comfortably at a bit more than shoulder width; knees bent; back straight; buttocks over your heels. If you feel any pain, the squat is too deep; straighten your knees a bit.

- Bend your elbows and place your arms in front of your chest, fingertips touching.
- As you look straight ahead, relax your shoulders, keeping your head erect.
- Let your elbows drop to a level that is comfortable and feel the gentle elongation of your neck. Imagine that the top of your head is connected to the ceiling by a cord that is pulling it up.
- Tighten your buttocks and lift your pelvic floor. Squeeze your butt muscles, lifting internally. Imagine that you are trying to draw your anus as close to your belly button as you can. Hold this posture as long as you comfortably can. Thirty seconds is a good start. Teachers of t'ai chi, from which this posture is derived, advise holding it for 10 minutes.
- Do not hold your breath. Breathe slowly, and follow the movement of your breath. As you inhale, air will flow through your nostrils and fill the bottom of your lungs. If your

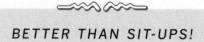

BETTER THAN SIT-UPS!

Did you know that sit-ups and crunches are actually *not* the best exercise for strengthening and toning your abs? Four muscles sheath your abdomen: rectus, transversus, internal oblique, and external oblique. Sit-ups and crunches work only the rectus muscle, the one that covers the front of your abdomen. But when the rectus gets tight and firm, it actually shortens your waistline—and it does little to stabilize your spine.

The transversus, on the other hand, is like a natural corset. When it gets tight and firm, this muscle draws in and elongates your waistline while protecting your lower back. The Wood-Chopping Exercise I recommend is the best there is for toning your transversus. You can perform it even if you are seriously overweight—just start slow and build up gradually.

breathing is relaxed, your chest will barely move. Instead, your diaphragm will flatten and your belly will push out—the so-called "belly breathing" that can be very helpful in managing stress. (For more on stress, see Chapter 8.)

2. WOOD-CHOPPING EXERCISE

- Stand with your feet a bit more than shoulder width apart.
- Raise your arms over your head, fingers intertwined. Pull your arms upward and to the right, as if reaching up to swing an axe.
- Slowly swing your hands down in an arc toward your left knee, as if chopping a log in slow motion. You don't need to bend very deeply at the waist, and you should feel no strain on your back. (If your back hurts, bend less.) Keep your feet planted firmly on the floor. Don't lock your knees—they should bend ever so slightly.
- When you've brought your hands as low as you comfortably can alongside your left leg, slowly swing them upward and to your right in an arc, the opposite movement of the wood chop.
- Breathe out during the downward swing (the chop) and breathe in during the upward swing (the reverse chop). Allow each swing to take 6 seconds to complete.
- After completing a cycle of 12 chops and 12 reverse chops, change sides: draw your hands over your head and to the left, and swing down toward your right knee.

FOR EXTRA CREDIT:
- If you can comfortably do a series of twelve cycles on each side, add some weight by holding a ball in your hands. A rubber kick ball is good for a start. As you get stronger, you can move up to a weighted medicine ball. If you work out at a gym, you can use a weight machine with handles

and pulleys (but then you have to set up the chop and reverse chops separately).

3. SHOULDER STRETCH CIRCLES

WARM-UP:
- Complete either the Serenity Crouch or the Wood-Chopping Exercise.

THE EXERCISE:
- Stand comfortably with your feet a bit more than shoulder width apart and your knees slightly bent. Relax your shoulders.
- Stretch your right arm out in front of you, palm down, and gently swing it back up over your head in a complete arc, forming a backward circle. Allow your arm to relax and your elbow to bend as you make the circle. Do 10 of these.
- Reverse direction and do 10 forward circles.
- Repeat 10 forward and 10 backward circles with your left arm.

4. SHOULDER STRENGTH CIRCLES

WARM-UP:
- Complete the Shoulder Stretch Circles.

THE EXERCISE:
- Extend both arms in front of you, parallel to the floor, palms down. Hold them in that position as you make small circles in the air with your hands. Make 10 small circles with your right hand moving clockwise and your left hand moving counterclockwise.
- Make 10 more circles with your left hand moving clockwise and your right hand moving counterclockwise.
- Now, without lowering your arms, extend them out to the

sides, perpendicular to your body. Make 20 small circles in the air with your hands—10 backward and then 10 forward.

- Without lowering your arms, bring them back in front of you, extended, palms up, and make 20 circles in the air with each hand, 10 clockwise and 10 counterclockwise.
- Without lowering your arms, extend them out to your sides, palms upward, and make 10 backward and then 10 forward circles.
- Without lowering your arms, stretch them out in front of you, parallel to the floor.
- Raise your arms straight up over your head, palms facing each other, and stretch them up toward the ceiling. Let your shoulders relax downward while keeping your arms extended upward.
- Do 20 circles with your hands, 10 in each direction.
- Slowly lower your arms to stretch them out in front of you, parallel to the floor, palms down.

You have just completed one full shoulder cycle. When you finish, you should feel warmth flowing through the shoulder muscles. When you can do one cycle without feeling any strain, gradually work your way up to three full cycles without stopping.

FOR EXTRA STRENGTH:
- When you can do three cycles without feeling any strain, try doing the series with a small weight in each hand, starting with 1 pound and gradually working your way up to 3 pounds.

NOTE: When professional football players do this exercise, they use only 5 to 10 pounds in each hand.

5. HAMSTRING STRETCH

PREPARATION:
- Have a towel or a rubber exercise band nearby.

HOW ARE YOUR HAMSTRINGS?

Your hamstrings are the straplike muscles that run along the back of your thighs. There are two common hamstring problems. One is having hamstrings that are too weak, compared to your quadriceps (the muscles that run along the front of your thighs), which puts excess pressure on your knees. The Knee Protector exercise can help with that imbalance.

The second common problem is excessively tight hamstrings, which limits flexible movement of the lower back. Check out your hamstrings by lying on the floor on your back, resting comfortably on a thick carpet or mat. With one leg stretched straight along the floor, slowly raise the other leg, keeping your knee straight and pointing your raised foot toward the ceiling. With healthy hamstring flexibility, you can, without assistance, bring your raised leg perpendicular to the floor, at about a 90-degree angle, keeping your leg straight. Most people get stuck between 45 and 60 degrees.

This is also the best position for stretching your hamstrings. Many exercise trainers and yoga instructors ask their clients to stretch their hamstrings in a standing position, but unless you're a trained dancer, you can't really stretch your hamstrings when standing. When you're standing, your hamstrings are always contracted to some extent, in order to stabilize your upright posture. The standing hamstring stretch mostly succeeds in stretching the ligaments of the lower back, a harmful rather than beneficial activity. So lie on your back, on the floor, to stretch your hamstrings, using my Hamstring Stretch.

THE EXERCISE:
- Lie comfortably on your back, one leg straight out on the floor, the other raised straight up, pointing toward the ceiling.
- Place the towel or exercise band behind the calf or ankle of your raised leg, holding one end in each hand.

- Breathe out slowly, relax, and pull on the towel or band gently and steadily, keeping your knee straight and raising your leg as close to a 90-degree angle from the floor as you comfortably can. *Don't overstretch.* There should be no pain or discomfort. A gentle stretch every day is the only way to improve flexibility.
- Hold the stretch for at least 60 seconds.
- Repeat with your other leg.

6. HAMSTRING STRENGTHENER

PREPARATION:
- Have a chair nearby.

THE EXERCISE:
- Lie on your back on the floor, comfortably supported by a thick rug, mat, or pillow. Position a chair about 2 feet in front of your buttocks. The leg you are not exercising should lie alongside the edge of the chair.
- Raise the other leg and place its heel on the chair seat.
- Bear down steadily on the chair seat, pushing your heel toward the floor. This action contracts the hamstring.
- Hold this contraction for 15 seconds. *Remember to keep breathing.* Do not hold your breath.
- Repeat this contraction with your other leg.
- Complete a set of 8 contractions with each leg.

If you have knee problems, do the following Knee Protector exercise.

7. KNEE PROTECTOR

PREPARATION:
- Have a towel handy.

- Sit on the floor with your legs stretched out straight in front of you.
- Roll up the towel like a log and place it under the back of your right knee. Your leg remains extended on the floor.
- Point the toes of your right foot in the direction of your head.
- Tighten the front of your thighs and press the back of your knee firmly against the rolled-up towel, as if you were using your knee to flatten the towel against the floor. (Touch your thighs to check yourself: the muscle with the greatest tension should be the one on the inside of the thigh just above the knee.) Hold this contraction for 15 seconds.
- Repeat with the other leg.
- Complete a set of 8 contractions with each leg.

Keep Moving!

Once you've started losing weight and feeling more fit, you may want to start engaging in more strenuous recreational exercise or working out at a gym. Here's a hint: find something that you enjoy. There's no better motivation to keep moving than the pleasure you get from doing it. Gym workouts, tennis, softball, basketball, dance, swimming—find one or more activities you enjoy, and then find ways to build them into your day. But don't stop walking—and don't give up your core strengtheners and knee protectors. The more active you are, the more you'll need them.

As I think about the joy of movement, I'm reminded of my patient Marie. Although Marie had been physically active most of her life—a runner in her twenties and thirties, a practitioner of t'ai chi in her early forties—she had gotten out of the habit of exercise in her late forties and had gradually

LITTLE BY LITTLE: HOW EVEN SMALL AMOUNTS OF EXERCISE ADD UP

Your *basal metabolic rate (BMR)* is the minimum amount of energy your body burns each minute, as measured in calories. The least amount of energy you can burn—your BMR—is what your body uses to stay alive while you're lying down or sleeping. From this baseline, any kind of physical activity, even sitting up, increases the number of calories you're burning.

  • **Activities that raise your caloric expenditure by about 50 percent over your BMR:** reading; working at a desk, computer, or laboratory bench; watching TV; playing cards or video games; sewing; playing a musical instrument while seated
  • **Activities that raise your caloric expenditure by about 150 percent over your BMR:** preparing food; standing at a desk or laboratory bench; ironing; playing a musical instrument or arcade games while standing
  • **Activities that raise your caloric expenditure by about 250 percent over your BMR:** walking at a moderate pace (3 miles an hour or less) on level ground; housecleaning; carpentry, plumbing, or electrical work; working in a garage or restaurant; taking care of young children; playing golf, baseball, or Ping-Pong; sailing
  • **Activities that raise your caloric expenditure by about 450 percent over your BMR:** walking at a brisk pace (over 3 miles an hour) on level ground or walking uphill at any pace; gardening; cycling; skiing; playing tennis; dancing; carrying a heavy load of any type
  • **Activities that raise your caloric expenditure by about 750 percent over your BMR:** running or jogging; mountain biking; walking uphill while carrying a load; climbing; cutting down trees; heavy digging; playing strenuous sports like football, basketball, or soccer

(Continued)

Note that the greatest relative jump in caloric output comes when you replace sitting with standing. I don't recommend staying on your feet all day—you'll get a lot more pleasure out of moving than standing still! But I do want you to see how even very little shifts in your activity level can help burn calories and speed up your metabolism. And the less active you've been, the more difference even a little change will make. Of course, your ultimate goal isn't so much burning calories as healing inflammation. But there's no reason you can't do both!

put on weight. She noticed a distinct vicious cycle: the less she moved, the more weight she gained; the more weight she gained, the less she felt like moving. By the time she came to me, she felt discouraged by both her weight and her lethargy.

I suggested to her that she start small—in her case, a twenty-minute walk five days a week. Marie had a demanding job, and she often ate in restaurants—so she decided to build in a short walk as part of her lunch or dinner break. "Walking to a restaurant doesn't seem like it's going to do much for my weight," she warned me, but I told her to give it a try.

Sure enough, within two weeks, Marie was ready to take on a thirty-minute walk, and the following month, a forty-minute walk. She noticed the weight-loss benefits within the first two weeks as her clothes started to fit differently. But more important to her was the boost in energy and morale. "I really feel like I've gotten my city back," she told me. "I hadn't realized how much I had come to dread even having to walk the few blocks from my house to the subway, or how much I'd come to depend on cabs to go even a few blocks. Now, I enjoy walking from one place to another, and I feel freer and more powerful—as though I can go anywhere, do anything. I can't believe what a big difference something so small has made."

FRUIT SPRITZERS

Deep blue, ruby red, rich purple; colorful, sweet, a little tangy—nonalcoholic fruit spritzers are a delicious and healthy beverage. They are refreshing, contain no alcohol, and have no added sugar or artificial sweeteners. No wonder they're a favorite of Dr. Galland! He's always stocking up on sparkling water and fruit concentrates and mixing up a new concoction with great flavor. It's a wonderful way to get antioxidants into a pleasant drink.

The recipe for a fruit spritzer is simple: Pour sparkling water over ice in a tall glass, add a little juice concentrate or juice, and mix well. Add a squeeze of lemon or lime for some refreshing tartness.

Basic Ingredients for a Fruit Spritzer

8 ounces sparkling mineral water or seltzer
Ice
2 tablespoons fruit juice concentrate such as pomegranate, cherry, blueberry or ¼ cup of your favorite fruit juice
Slice of lemon or lime

Spritzers are a really good alternative to soft drinks and alcoholic beverages. In fact, everyone in the family will enjoy creating their own special varieties of these kid-friendly drinks.

Summary of Chapter Seven: The Joy of Movement: How Exercise Can Help You Overcome Leptin Resistance

1. Even a slight increase in physical activity can benefit your health.
2. Physical activity of any kind burns calories, strengthens muscles, combats aging, and improves your mood.
3. Moderate physical activity reduces inflammation.
4. Moderate physical activity helps reverse leptin resistance, enabling you to lose weight.

eight

~~~~~

Relaxing into a Healthy Weight

Ginger was a forty-two-year-old realtor who came to see me because of her strong family history of diabetes and high blood pressure. Fortunately, she hadn't yet been diagnosed with these conditions, but she was concerned that her increasing weight would make her more susceptible to them, a prospect that she found particularly disturbing because she'd seen how grievously her mother's health and quality of life had deteriorated under the burden of these two illnesses.

"Over the years my weight just kept climbing," Ginger told me—from 130 when she was married at age twenty-five to 170 now, seventeen years later. "Every so often, I'd diet like crazy, drop a few pounds—and then start gaining again."

Ginger had learned a lot about nutrition as she'd helped her mother cope with her health problems, so she grasped the principles of the Fat Resistance Diet right away. When I told her that adult-onset diabetes and high blood pressure were both related to chronic inflammation, my program made even more sense to her.

But as Ginger shared more details about her life, I began to suspect that even the best diet in the world would not be enough to heal her inflammation without some additional help. Between her work and her family, she was busy all the time, and almost continually overwhelmed with stress. "If I'm lucky, I get six hours of sleep," she told me. "Most nights, it's more like five." And as for her waking hours, most of them were spent, as she put it, "playing beat the clock." Even Ginger's exercise program was "beat the clock"—a frantic forty minutes each morning on a stationary bicycle, while she made memos to herself on a portable tape recorder and fielded questions from her husband and kids.

Not surprisingly, Ginger felt more or less continually fatigued, which made it difficult for her to eat well or exercise. And she was extremely susceptible to illness, catching every virus that came around.

After Ginger finished describing her daily schedule, I sat for a moment, trying to find a way to explain the problem. "Look," I finally said, "managing your lifestyle is just as important as managing your diet. Is there any part of your day when you just get to kick back and relax?"

Ginger shook her head.

"Is there any part of your day when you just—enjoy yourself?"

Ginger shook her head again. "I know it's not good, the way I live . . ." Her voice trailed off.

"It's not a question of good or bad," I said. "When you don't get enough sleep and when you're constantly stressed, you're literally changing your biology. Both stress and sleep deprivation stimulate your adrenal glands—not temporarily, to meet a single challenge, but continually. So instead of one shot of cortisol, the stress hormone, you get a fairly continuous dose."

Excess cortisol has a number of different effects on the body, I continued, but the bottom line is that lack of sleep and sustained psychological stress can contribute to inflammation and leptin resistance. No matter how good her diet was, I told Ginger, she wouldn't be able to lose weight permanently by simply changing what she ate. If she really wanted to avoid her mother's fate, she had to find a way to live a calmer, more pleasurable life—and to get at least seven hours of sleep every night. "Now," I concluded, "let's see if we can figure out how to build more sleep into your life—and more fun."

Ginger began to protest. She had kids to take care of, a job to perform, a household to run.

"Remember," I added, "de-stressing is essential for healing inflammation and overcoming leptin resistance. And until you've resolved your leptin resistance, you'll have an extremely hard time losing weight."

"All right," Ginger said slowly. "Maybe I could cut out watching the eleven o'clock news. That way I could maybe get to bed before midnight. And that would give me another hour's sleep."

"That sounds like a good beginning," I said. "Let's start there."

Ginger wasn't always able to get enough sleep, but the next time I saw her, she had made a definite improvement in her sleep schedule—and found that she functioned better as a result. "I'm actually more efficient," she admitted. "I might as well get the sleep—I can get more done that way."

With her sleep problem on the way to a solution, I asked Ginger to give herself the gift of some quiet time each day. Once she learned the secret of deep relaxation, she would be able to use it for support on a daily basis. I instructed her in a simple technique that I had first taught to my patients more than twenty-five years ago (a technique that I explain on page 154).

Ginger found that spending five minutes twice a day with this technique was not only relaxing but refreshing and gave her renewed energy and focus, so that it was easier for her to meet her responsibilities. It proved especially useful when she felt stressed and was tempted to calm herself by eating, or if she was having a hard time falling asleep at night.

Over the year that I saw her, Ginger achieved a slow but steady weight loss—twenty-five pounds so far—and found herself really enjoying the Fat Resistance Diet's emphasis on fresh fruits, vegetables, spices, and herbs. She also became markedly more relaxed and alert, thanks to both the sleep and the relaxation that she was now building into each day.

"I hate to say it, but I actually get *more* done this way," she confessed the last time I saw her. "I handle situations better—especially when they involve conflict, which believe me, there's a lot of in my business. I make fewer mistakes and get into fewer arguments. And when I find myself getting snappish over little things, I know what to do to step back and calm down." She shook her head in disbelief. "I *really* didn't expect to get this from a medical doctor, but I've got to admit it: these days, life is more fun."

Cortisol: How Stress Makes You Fat

One of our most important stress hormones is cortisol, a chemical produced by your adrenal glands when your body, mind, and emotions all need to gear up to meet a significant challenge. If you've got a pressing deadline or a sick child, cortisol goes coursing through your bloodstream as you mobilize to take care of business.

Ideally, you'd release cortisol only in the face of a specific, temporary challenge—the old "fight or flight" reaction that occurs in response to a particular danger. Ideally, too, the period of relaxation and calm that followed your response to the challenge would give your body an opportunity to "come down" from your cortisol high and rebalance your biochemistry.

But so many of us are living with continual high- or even low-grade stress that our cortisol levels never have a chance to rebalance. And when you consider that one of the stressors that promotes the release of cortisol is inflammation, you can see how the vicious cycle of obesity and inflammation continues—because, among its other attributes, cortisol actually encourages your body to hold on to its fat.[2] In our modern world, common sources of chronic stress are likely to include overwork, lack of sleep, and environmental toxins (see Chapter 9) as well as inflammation. Cortisol actually causes fat cells to grow, and the presence of this hormone will increase your amount of belly fat in particular. The weight gain that results once again produces more inflammation—and a new vicious cycle begins.

Elevated cortisol levels can cause a number of other serious problems, including

- fluid retention
- muscle weakness
- memory loss
- high blood pressure
- osteoporosis
- elevated blood sugar levels

The associated increase in blood sugar is especially problematic, as it stimulates a further increase in insulin—and, as we saw in Chapters 5 and 6, if you are overweight your insulin levels may be too high.[3] So as you can see, the inflammation-cortisol connection wreaks havoc with important hormones that regulate the metabolism of your fat cells—insulin and cortisol itself—in addition to setting up the fat-inducing condition known as leptin resistance. As you may have guessed, one major solution to all these problems is to heal your inflammation with the Fat Resistance Diet.

SLEEP AND WEIGHT LOSS

Among its many other benefits, adequate sleep is crucial to achieving and maintaining a healthy weight. Two recent studies indicate that people who slept five hours or less each night had higher levels of *ghrelin*, a hormone produced by the stomach that stimulates appetite.[1] At the same time, sleep deprivation lowered the subjects' leptin levels—and leptin, you'll recall, is a hormone that suppresses appetite. So if you deprive yourself of the sleep you need, you'll find yourself hungrier—and probably heavier.

I don't want to leave you with a negative impression of corti-sol, which your body desperately needs. A deficiency of cortisol can have disastrous results: severe fatigue, low blood pressure, the inability to tolerate stress, and an impairment to your immunity that is also associated with a tendency to unchecked inflammation. Low levels of cortisol may explain why some people develop au-toimmune disorders like rheumatoid arthritis.

But excess cortisol can be equally damaging. Animal studies suggest that cortisol contributes to leptin resistance, perhaps by supporting the SOCS-3 counterinflammatory response (see Chapter 2).[4] Cortisol also turns off the adiponectin gene, reducing the level of this beneficial hormone.[5] And both animal and human studies indicate that cortisol increases food consumption by turn-ing off the brain's other natural appetite-suppressing signals. Since leptin resistance has a similar effect, you can see why high levels of cortisol give you a double or even a triple whammy: in-flammation, cortisol, and leptin resistance are all interacting with one another and with obesity to boost your appetite, disrupt your metabolism, and produce an even greater weight gain.[6]

So the solution, as I explained to Ginger, is threefold:

1. Combat inflammation at the cellular level with the Fat Resistance Diet.
2. Combat both inflammation and stress with exercise (see Chapter 7).
3. Combat stress directly by getting sufficient sleep, building in time for relaxation, and using stress-management techniques to help you stay serene and focused.

Managing Your Stress

When Ginger and I were discussing the punishing stress levels in her life, she burst out, "But *how* do I de-stress? Every time I try to relax, I just get more tense."

STRESS REDUCERS

• **Take a walk.** A brisk walk or a leisurely stroll—even one as short as five minutes—gets your muscles moving and refreshes your mind. If you're feeling stressed at work, getting away from the problem—or simply away from your desk—can be an efficient way to solve the problem as well as a terrific de-stressing device.

• **Soak in the tub.** If you can find twenty minutes somewhere in your day to simply shut the bathroom door and immerse yourself in a warm bath, you'll be giving yourself not only a wonderful treat but also a significant boost to your weight-loss efforts. Find some sensory cues—soft lighting and music—that enable you to shift gears from "doing" to "being." Epsom salts in the bathwater help to relax your muscles.

• **Bathe your feet.** If you don't have time for an entire bath, try soaking your feet for five minutes or so in a tub or basin of warm water. Find a comfortable sitting or reclining posture, immerse your feet, and close your eyes. If it's a hot day, you might prefer to soak in cool or room-temperature water, which will help bring down your body temperature. For maximum benefit, breathe slowly and focus entirely on your breath and your bodily sensations, letting go of all your chores and obligations.

• **Listen to music.** I don't mean put on some background music that only raises the noise level in your home or workplace, but rather, choose some music that you love and allow yourself anywhere from five to thirty minutes to simply listen to it. Find a listening mode, whether headphones or speakers, that allows you to isolate yourself from all other demands, so that you can shut your eyes, quiet your mind, and simply allow the music to work its calming magic. Even if you've chosen a hard-driving rock CD or an intense piece of classical music, you'll find yourself relaxing as you focus on the music rather than on your numerous work and family tasks. Your goal is to quiet your mind and allow your muscles to relax—and immersing yourself in the world of a song or symphony is one of the best ways to do that.

• **Connect to nature.** If you're lucky enough to live near trees, a beach, or open fields, find a way to put yourself in touch with the sights, sounds, and smells of the natural world. Alternatively, concentrate for five minutes on a favorite plant or a vase of lovely flowers. Again, your goal is to quiet your mind, so give yourself something on which you can focus that allows you to switch your mind-set—from *doing* to simply *appreciating*.

• **Spend some time in a garden.** If you've got a patch of vegetables or flowers in your own backyard, pulling some weeds or standing quietly with a hose can be terrifically therapeutic. Even five minutes spent gardening can relax your mind and refresh your spirit.

• **Prepare food.** For many of my patients, the quiet, peaceful act of working with food can be a meditative experience—calmly chopping carrots, assembling ingredients for a salad, carefully arranging fruits and vegetables on a plate. If you do a lot of mental work during the day, you might find it therapeutic to engage in a more physical, hands-on type of activity.

• **Get a massage.** This option requires more time, money, and commitment than the others on the list—but I can't recommend it too strongly. Not only are the health benefits of massage well documented, but the relaxation benefits are obvious.

I saw her point. Seeing relaxation as an obligation or a goal pretty much defeats its purpose. I thought for a moment and then offered her an alternative definition of relaxation: *quieting the mind.*

Think about what it's usually like "inside your head." If you're like most of us, you experience a constant stream of mental chatter: "Don't forget to the pay the electric bill. OK, I'll call Helen back, but not today—tomorrow. I wonder if Joe will remember to pick the kids up from school, or if I should call to remind him?" For many of us, the only way to silence the chatter is by distracting ourselves—with TV, background music, phone calls, email, video games, reading, other conversations, or plunging more deeply into an absorbing task. But none of these distractions—pleasurable or useful as they may be—really address the mental chatter; they only shift it to another topic.

Meditation and meditative movement—whether yoga, t'ai chi, swimming, stretching, or some other form of movement that requires full concentration—are about creating a profound silence within the mind. This silence is deeply relaxing and restorative, and it's one of the best antistress devices I know. A number of different disciplines offer approaches to quieting the chatter in the mind and achieving deep relaxation, and I invited Ginger to explore them at her leisure. Meanwhile, I offered her the following introduction to quieting the mind and relaxing the body, which I hoped would pave the way for whatever else she might want to do:

- Sit in a comfortable chair with a straight back and good back support. Let your feet rest flat on the floor while your hands rest on your thighs, with your arms falling comfortably by your sides.
- Gently draw your shoulders down toward the floor. Feel the stretch in the muscle that connects your neck and shoulders (the trapezius). Massage it for a few moments, if you like, to help it relax. Recognize how much tension was in that muscle before you lowered your shoulders. Now relax your shoulders and let them settle into a natural position. Notice how much lower they are now than before you stretched them downward.
- Gently stretch your fingers along your thighs, as if you were trying to wrap them around your leg. Then relax the stretch of your hands and let your fingers rest comfortably. Observe how much tension existed in your hands before this stretch.
- Without opening your mouth or parting your lips, draw your jaw downward, toward your chest. Then relax your jaw. Feel how far it has dropped and how the tension in your jaw muscles has slackened. Pay attention to the position of your tongue. Allow it to float easily in your mouth,

without pressing against the roof or the floor. You may notice an increase in the flow of saliva, a sign of relaxation that makes this a good exercise to perform before a meal.

- Imagine that a gentle hand is smoothing your forehead, relaxing the furrows of your brow. Imagine the hand traveling over the top of your head and down the back of your neck, relaxing each muscle it touches with its caress. This brings your attention back to your shoulders.
- Run through this set of stretches and images one more time.
- Observe your breath. Feel the air pass in through your nostrils and down the back of your throat. Place one hand on your chest and one hand on your belly. This breath should not fill your chest, because it is a relaxed breath, not a deep full breath. Instead, when you breathe in, your belly should move outward as the diaphragm pushes down. This is sometimes called belly breathing—the calmest form of breathing. Chest breathing is only for exertion, so if you find that your chest rises and your abdomen flattens when you breathe in, see if you can reverse the breathing pattern so that your chest stays still and your belly expands.
- One more time, relax your jaw and tongue. Imagine once again the gentle hand smoothing your forehead and caressing your head and neck.

Think of this little exercise as an excellent prelude to meditation, spiritual reflection, or prayer. It calms your sympathetic nervous system and is an excellent way to begin relaxing your body and mind. You can do it almost anywhere, as many times a day as you care to. Once you know it and have trained your breath, you can relax with it in as little as thirty seconds, but I encourage you to spend more time with it. In fact, when you've gotten used to doing it, try allowing yourself ten to fifteen minutes of observing your breath—at least once, just to see how it feels. I also encourage you to explore meditative techniques, which are the most ancient and successful approaches to stress management that we have.

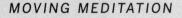

MOVING MEDITATION

Any kind of movement or exercise can be relaxing and help release stress. But the most profoundly relaxing and transformative exercise is that which combines "emptying the mind" and deep breathing with physical movement.

Western forms of activity, such as swimming, running, and modern dance, can serve as a kind of moving meditation, in which breath awareness is part of the activity and the mind is completely focused on how the body is moving. If you're thinking about your to-do list while swimming or running, you'll find the activity far less relaxing than if you empty your mind and simply focus on your physical self.

Eastern practices, especially yoga and t'ai chi, are also wonderfully effective ways to experience the profound silence that follows when you quiet your mind. These practices encourage participants to focus entirely on body and breath, allowing the mind's chatter to subside. Many of my patients have told me that they've become more creative, emotionally expressive, and "in touch with themselves" after only a few weeks of these practices, which I attribute to the restorative effects of quieting the mind. If you're looking for a way to enjoy movement and de-stress at the same time, consider taking a course in yoga, t'ai chi, or perhaps another martial art. You can confine yourself to a weekly or twice-weekly class, or develop your own daily practice of anywhere from five to forty-five minutes a day.

Restoring Joy Is Crucial for Your Health

As far as I'm concerned, the dangerous chemical imbalances that result from uninterrupted stress are as hazardous to your health as a diet consisting entirely of junk food or a periodic session of deep breathing behind the exhaust pipe of a bus. Stress and lack of sleep are seriously bad for you, and if you're interested in losing weight, you need to address these issues as much as your diet and exercise. The good news is, when you've made even a tiny change, both the emotional benefits and the improvement in your health are powerfully reinforcing, encouraging you to continue choosing ways to nourish and nurture your need for serenity and joy.

I've noticed with a number of my stressed-out patients that they're able to do almost anything that feels like a task—especially a task that is crucial for their health—but they have trouble finding the time to just "be." So let me put it in the strongest possible terms: *In my medical opinion, building in time to "be" and relax, finding ways to enjoy your life, and reconnecting to your quiet inner self are just as crucial for your long-term health as changing your diet and getting regular exercise.* As we've seen in this chapter, stress literally alters your biology. It causes weight gain, inflammation, and a host of other damaging effects that can become literally life-threatening. So being good to yourself is no more "optional" than a diabetic taking her insulin or a heart patient ceasing to smoke. Find a way to be good to yourself—and restore the joy your life was meant to have.

Summary of Chapter Eight: Relaxing into a Healthy Weight

1. Lack of sleep activates the hormone ghrelin, which causes feelings of hunger, and suppresses leptin, your most important fat-burning hormone.
2. The stress hormone cortisol, made by your adrenal glands, increases leptin resistance and the need to eat. Elevated cortisol also causes fluid retention, muscle weakness, memory loss, bone loss, high blood pressure, and high blood sugar.

AN HERB GARDEN

There is magic in a garden. It's a thrill to see sunlight and water make a little plant grow and spread its leaves. The beauty of nature rejuvenates and inspires.

The quiet thrill of gardening can be enjoyed by planting an herb garden in the kitchen, patio, or backyard. Herbs are great to grow in or near the kitchen so you can pick a few leaves while you're cooking. In fact, restaurant chefs often keep an herb garden near the kitchen. We use herbs in many of our recipes in the Fat Resistance Diet. I recommend having herbs every day, for their wonderful flavor and ability to reduce inflammation.

Fresh herbs are a great choice for indoors because you can plant them in fairly small pots, plus they're easy to grow. I like to plant basil, parsley, and cilantro. Follow the same simple steps I do, and you will be picking delicious fresh herbs in few days.

First, I pick up some clay pots and saucers, organic potting soil in a bag, and small starter plants at a garden center.

At home, I put a few pebbles into the bottom of the pots for drainage and place the pots on saucers. I fill the pots about ¾ full with potting soil. Then I carefully remove a little herb plant from its container, transfer it to the pot, and place soil all around the plant with my hands. You want to pack down the soil to give the plant a sturdy base. Sprinkle it with about 1 cup of water, and you're done.

Herbs seem to like a mixture of direct sun and some shade. Give them a little water each day to keep the soil moist, and move them into a shady spot if the leaves get burned by the sun. Nourished by your attention and care, your kitchen garden will be good to grow!

3. A period of deep relaxation once a day and a good night's sleep are major aids to weight loss.

4. The Fat Resistance Diet and lifestyle are designed to add joy, not deprivation, to your life. Joy is important for health and long-term weight control.

nine

〰〰〰

Detoxify—and Lose Weight

Amy had been struggling with asthma, fatigue, and weight gain since she'd first enrolled in nursing school some fifteen years earlier. She came to see me at age thirty-nine because of asthma and chronic fatigue. I immediately saw that she was also forty-five pounds overweight, despite long hours on her feet at her grueling job. "I've never been able to lose more than five pounds on any diet," she told me when I asked. "I've pretty much given up in that department."

All three of Amy's problems—asthma, fatigue, and weight gain—were related to inflammation, which I knew could be caused by a wide variety of factors, including environmental toxins. So I asked about her working conditions, and was interested to hear that at one of the hospitals she'd worked in after graduating, several staff members had fallen ill, at about the same time that Amy's asthma took a turn for the worse. The problem had been environmental—mold in an improperly ventilated operating room—which I knew could trigger asthmatic and allergic reactions.

Amy had eventually left her hospital work because of lung

problems. "Those chemical cleaners they use really got to me after a while," she explained. "So I went to work as a visiting nurse. But I ran into the same problems there—I'd walk into a house and start to get sick. Or maybe it wouldn't happen right away, but sooner or later, if I spent enough time in a house where someone used one of those real strong cleansers, my eyes would burn or I'd have trouble breathing." She was currently working in the office of an allergist, which provided a reasonably clean environment.

Amy's previous doctor had prescribed the standard medical treatment for her severe asthma attacks: inhalers and oral steroids (cortisone). These did help ease the attacks, but the steroids drove her weight up. "And whatever I gained, I could never lose again," Amy told me. "That was my new plateau. No matter how much I dieted, no matter how much I exercised. Of course, with the asthma, that wasn't much. But it didn't matter anyway. My weight just stayed up there."

As I considered Amy's condition, I could see the making of yet another vicious cycle. Inflammation—triggered by environmental factors or by Amy's obesity—was producing leptin resistance, even as her increased stores of fat were raising the levels of leptin in her blood. Leptin resistance made it difficult for her to lose her excess fat—and the excess leptin produced by the extra fat might be aggravating her asthmatic inflammation. (Even thin asthmatics have relatively high leptin levels.)[1] So I thought that if Amy could lose some weight, her health would improve on all fronts.

Unfortunately for Amy, just improving her diet—while crucial—would not be enough. Based on what she was telling me about her sensitivity to the hospital and home environments in which she had worked, her inflammation would not clear up until we were able to help reduce the total burden of toxins in her body.[2] We'd also have to prevent continual reexposure. Until we detoxified both her body and her surroundings, Amy would continue to struggle with asthma and obesity.

When I explained this analysis to Amy, she stared at me for a moment, then let out an enormous sigh of relief. "I'm just glad there's an explanation," she told me. "It was so awful, feeling like I was getting sicker and sicker and couldn't do anything about it."

Our first step, I told her, was to identify potential sources of toxins and allergens in her home, food, and water. Then, we had to figure out how to avoid those inflammatory triggers. Meanwhile, I would find a way to adapt the Fat Resistance Diet to her unique needs, so that it could begin to heal her inflammation as soon as possible without setting off further toxic responses. Finally, I'd suggest special foods and nutritional supplements to help Amy detoxify.

People like Amy who struggle with food allergies and environmental sensitivities have the most difficult time losing weight, perhaps because their inflammation is more severe, or perhaps because there are more factors to reinforce it. To her surprise and delight, Amy did lose weight on the Fat Resistance Diet—slowly, to be sure, but persistently. She lost ten pounds almost immediately, within the first month, and then another ten pounds over the subsequent year. The following year, she dropped another fifteen pounds; and she lost her final ten pounds during the next six months.

"It seems as though I'm losing weight more and more quickly," Amy commented, and I assured her that she was. As her body became less toxic, a healthy weight became easier to achieve. And indeed, for the past two years, Amy has maintained her goal weight, following her unique version of the Fat Resistance Diet and exercising for thirty to sixty minutes every day. Best of all, she no longer experiences any problems with asthma or fatigue.

How Toxins Increase Body Fat

We live in a world that seems tailor-made to produce inflammation. The food we eat, the water we drink, the air we breathe—even some of the furniture in our homes—can cause cellular damage that leads directly to chronic, low-grade inflammation. We shouldn't be surprised. If we keep our immune system constantly busy fending off toxic challenges, it's bound to become hypersensitive. This hair-trigger reactivity results in a slow, steady secretion of "pro-inflammatory cytokines"—chemicals that, as we saw in Chapter 2, trigger inflammation—the process that is supposed to drive out infection and heal the remaining tissue.

For some people—asthmatics and environmentally sensitive people like Amy—their hypersensitive immune systems begin to overrespond to potential threats. Dust, mold, and volatile chemicals like formaldehyde (found in many indoor environments) in sufficient quantity can provoke asthma even in healthy people; for people with asthma or other hypersensitivities, even a tiny exposure is amplified by the immune system. In your lungs, the swelling produced by the inflammatory response creates wheezing, shortness of breath, and, potentially, a full-blown asthma attack, which ironically is far more dangerous to the body than the threat that first provoked the inflammatory response.

A large body of research has shown that exposure to environmental toxins is a significant cause of the increasing worldwide epidemic of allergic diseases.[3] The chronic inflammation that results from toxic exposure may contribute to the development of autoimmune diseases and cancer. And, because the inflammatory response sets in motion the anti-inflammatory response, we can end up with leptin resistance and excess cortisol, both of which practically guarantee that we will become and remain obese.

In Chapter 2, I described the way the body responds to inflammatory triggers. First, there is an inflammatory response, then an anti-inflammatory counterresponse. This anti-inflammatory counterresponse is led by a group of chemicals inside your cells called SOCS—and SOCS activation is a key cause of leptin resistance. SOCS also shifts the body's immune response into a pattern that favors allergy. Significantly, allergic sensitivity and leptin resistance appear to have much in common, and recent research indicates that environmental toxins can contribute to both.

Researchers at the University of Quebec have demonstrated a correlation between organochlorine pollutants (which contaminate drinking water, human breast milk, meat, poultry, and seafood) and a slowing of the metabolic rate.[*] Since organochlorines are fat-soluble, they're stored in your body's fat cells—so when you start to lose weight, they're released from your fat into your bloodstream. The Quebec researchers found a direct relationship between the release of these toxins while overweight individuals were dieting and the slowing of metabolism that dieting seems to induce. It's not clear *how* toxins slow dieters' metabolism—but the tendency of organochlorine pesticides to promote inflammation is one likely connection.

For most of us, cleaning up our diets, exercising, de-stressing, and, eventually, losing weight is enough to heal our inflammation. But those who are environmentally sensitive may need to take another step: cleaning up our personal environments. If the fumes from synthetic carpeting, pressed-wood furniture, household and industrial cleaners, office products, and other environmental dangers continually stimulate an inflammatory response, all the healthy eating and exercise in the world may not solve the problem.

Controlling environmental toxicity is perhaps the most challenging aspect of reversing chronic inflammation, since so many of the sources of toxicity are outside our individual control. Some researchers have suggested that the relatively recent galloping obesity epidemic in the cities of India and China is due to the burgeoning problem of Asian urban pollution (in addition to the increased consumption of fat and empty calories that a Western lifestyle is bringing to the East). In the United States, where most people spend 90 percent of their time indoors, the major sources of environmental pollution are indoor chemicals released from cleaning solutions, construction and home furnishing materials, office machines, and myriad sources we never even think about. These toxic invaders hitchhike on dust particles—so dusty environments intensify your exposure to chemicals.

Moreover, our meats, fish, fruits, vegetables, and drinking water may be laced with toxins of various kinds, from industrial runoff, commercial fertilizer, commercial animal feed, pesticides, and a host of other environmental hazards. When we lose weight, toxins stored in our fat are released into our bloodstream, and, as the Canadian researchers demonstrated, threaten to stall our weight-loss efforts.

Our livers are given the substantial task of filtering the blood and removing any toxins that have found their way there. Fortunately, the superfoods at the heart of the Fat Resistance Diet are the best assistance your liver can get for removing environmental toxins from your body: there is no better diet for detoxification.[5] Of course, the whole process works better if you can find a way to avoid putting the toxins back in!

ASTHMA, INFLAMMATION, AND YOUR WEIGHT

A number of factors seem to be associated with the development of asthma, including pollution (especially in cities)[6] and a dietary deficiency of vitamin C, omega-3 fats, selenium, and magnesium[7]—all nutrients that you lack when you don't eat enough fish, fruits, and vegetables. Put another way, the Fat Resistance Diet is the exact opposite of the type of diet that produces asthma, suggesting that the Fat Resistance Diet—rich in vitamins, minerals, and omega-3s—might be helpful to asthmatics. Although there is no research to support this contention, my clinical experience has borne it out.

Moreover, animal studies have shown that SOCS-3—the anti-inflammatory molecule that is a major cause of leptin resistance—also increases the occurrence of asthma and other allergic disorders.[8] Once again, the Fat Resistance Diet, with its anti-inflammatory properties, might reduce your body's need for SOCS-3—and so reduce your likelihood of asthma attacks.

The connection between toxicity and weight retention is borne out by my own clinical experience. Among my patients, those with the greatest difficulty losing weight seem to be people with severe sensitivity to the environment, including food allergies and food intolerances. So if you suffer from asthma, food allergies, or environmental sensitivity, then you, like Amy, must be especially careful about the toxins in your daily life. The good news is that because most of your exposure is likely from indoor toxins, you have a real opportunity to control this exposure, especially at home.

Cleansing Your Body and Your Environment: A Step-by-Step Approach

If you, like Amy, are suffering from environmental sensitivity, or if you suspect that toxic exposure is playing a role in your weight gain, asthma, or allergies, here's the detoxification program that I recommend.

STEP 1: IDENTIFY AND REMOVE THE POSSIBLE SOURCES OF TOXINS IN YOUR DIET AND ENVIRONMENT

Dust and chemical cleansers are two of the most common home-based sources of toxic invaders. Mold is another, encouraged by dampness, including the high humidity that can come from a humidifier. In Amy's case, I had to ask her to stop humidifying her bedroom and to remove the mold from her bathroom. She began to use an air purifier in her bedroom and a dehumidifier in her basement.

If you think your diet might be the problem, try this classic dietary elimination and challenge test. For five days, totally avoid a food that you usually eat every day. Then eat it again and notice how it affects your breathing, energy, and tendency to retain fluid. The most common food sensitivities causing inflammation and resistance to weight loss are wheat, milk, corn, soy, yeast, chocolate, and eggs, so if you're concerned about sensitivities, you might begin by testing for those. The Fat Resistance Diet is easy to modify, so you can easily develop a version of the diet that is free of milk or other dairy products, soy, wheat, corn, or any other component of concern. If you're allergic to fish and have to avoid it, you should increase your use of flaxseeds or take flax oil (about a tablespoon a day) to boost your omega-3 intake, as I described in Chapter 6.

Some people are sensitive to food additives and preservatives, so if you think you might be suffering from an intolerance to those substances, you can again perform a food elimination test to find out. The Fat Resistance Diet works fine with all organic and natural foods, so you shouldn't have any problem there.

STEP 2: DETOXIFY YOUR BODY

Amy detoxed herself by avoiding the dairy products to which she seemed to be particularly sensitive, and by making an effort to eat only whole, organic foods without additives, preservatives, or pesticides. She also engaged in vigorous exercise to help herself sweat—an excellent way to release toxins through the skin.

STEP 3: ADD SPECIAL FOODS TO YOUR DIET

Your major detox organ is your liver, so if you're trying to rid your body of accumulated poisons, you want to give your liver as much support as possible. Here are some special foods that are excellent supplements to the usual Fat Resistance Diet. Consider adding them for additional liver support:

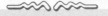

DETOX DECEPTION

There are many misconceptions floating around about detoxification, not to mention scores of books advocating detox for weight loss, general health, or both. Almost everything I've seen, however, misses the fundamental point: you don't need to detoxify your body, because your body detoxifies itself, naturally and automatically. If it didn't, you'd be dead in about six hours. What you can do, however, is ensure that the process is working smoothly.

Detoxification, like all other bodily processes, is primarily driven by enzymes, especially those in the liver, intestines, kidneys, lungs, and skin. These enzymes depend upon proteins, vitamins, minerals, and perhaps also flavonoids and carotenoids. So in order to keep your natural detox process functioning smoothly, what you really need is a healthy diet. In fact, you need precisely those vitamins, minerals, and phytonutrients that the Fat Resistance Diet is designed to provide.

In my opinion, the Fat Resistance Diet is the only detox diet you'll ever need. If you're really concerned about detox, I suggest you follow this diet closely and, to the extent that you can, avoid exposing yourself to the toxins that appear in your food and environment. Buy clean, organic foods; follow the detox suggestions that conclude this chapter; and make time for relaxation every day. I do not recommend fasting for detoxification, as I've seen many patients whose health deteriorated severely after several days of juice fasting; some suffered from gastrointestinal problems, fatigue, and food intolerance for weeks or even months afterward. The popular detox diets in the marketplace, which rely upon "cleansers" and fasts, pose a serious risk of depleting your liver—your major detox organ. Your liver needs significant nutritional support to do its job, relying upon enzymes and amino acids (derived from protein) to function, as well as zinc, selenium, and magnesium. Please don't starve this vital organ of the nutrients it needs, and stick to the nutritional prescriptions outlined in these pages.

- *Broccoli sprouts:* especially rich in a phytonutrient called sulforaphane, which stimulates the liver to make more detoxifying enzymes. If you can't find broccoli sprouts in a local market or health food store, you can make them yourself from broccoli seeds. Sprout the seeds for three days and add a handful to salad once a day.
- *Sea vegetables, especially those used in Japanese food:* hijiki, nori, wakame, dulse, and kelp are especially rich in anti-inflammatory carotenoids—and add exotic flavors in salads and as condiments.
- *Dark greens, such as kale, collards, dandelion greens, mustard greens, and Swiss chard:* these are loaded not only with carotenoids but with other phytonutrients that aid liver detoxification.

In Amy's case, I also recommended a multivitamin and mineral supplement that supplied her with folic acid (800 micrograms/day), selenium (200 micrograms/day) and magnesium (200 milligrams/day), all of which are important for detoxification processes. (For more on supplements, see Chapter 6.)

A Toxin-Free Home for Weight Loss and Health

One of the best things you can do for yourself—and your family—is to make your home as toxin-free as possible. Here are nine steps you can take to create a healthy home.*

1. Don't smoke and don't allow others to smoke in your home.
2. Remove your shoes when entering your home, a sensible habit used for centuries in Japan and Turkey. The dust tracked into your home on the soles of your shoes is

*Adapted from *Power Healing,* by Leo Galland, M.D. (Random House, 1998).

usually loaded with lead and pesticides and settles into carpets, where it can reside for years, rising up into the air you breathe.

3. Control moisture and its damage. High humidity, condensation, and leaks create conditions that favor mold growth. Watch for telltale signs like dampness, peeling paint, and discoloration—and don't delay correcting the problem.

4. Clean your refrigerator every week. Refrigerators are damp, dark, and packed with food, which makes them a haven for mold. Store cooked food for no more than two days before throwing it out. If you spot mold on cooked food, soft food, or juice, throw it all away— do not attempt to salvage any of it. If you see mold on the surface of an uncooked hard food like an apple, broccoli, cauliflower, hard cheese, onion, or potato, you can cut away an inch in every direction and use the remainder of the food, as long as you use it the same day.

5. Keep a carbon monoxide detector in the kitchen and bedrooms, and on every stair landing; vent all appliances to the outside, wherever possible.

6. Test for formaldehyde from time to time with a home testing kit. Formaldehyde is an irritating gas given off by pressed wood and finished plywood, new fabrics and carpeting, fresh paint and varnish (especially the water-soluble type), and various sprays and personal care products. If high levels are found, try to eliminate, ventilate, or cover the source. The most likely sources of high formaldehyde levels are particleboard, new carpets, and building materials.

7. Use environmentally friendly household products and cleaning solutions (see Resources). Don't store solvents in your kitchen or living area, even in closets.

8. Filter your tap water. Chlorination of municipal water

supplies produces potentially harmful substances called trihalomethanes (THMs), one reason that drinking more water has been associated with bladder and colon cancer in some studies. A charcoal filter helps to reduce these risks substantially.

BROCCOLI

Widely available in supermarkets, versatile, and easy to prepare, broccoli is my perfect go-to vegetable. Broccoli has become a classic American accompaniment to main dishes such as grilled salmon or roast chicken. This wonderful vegetable is equally at home in Italian cuisine, often sautéed with garlic, and in Asian dishes such as stir-fries.

Broccoli is part of the cruciferous vegetable family, chosen for their amazing health benefits for wide use in the Fat Resistance Diet. I'm excited to share with you how I enjoy broccoli.

Buying. Look for a bright green color and very firm stems. I like to buy organic broccoli when it's available.

Cooking. Cut off and discard the large main stem, then cut the broccoli into florets. Toss these into a strainer and rinse well with cold water. Transfer to a saucepan with 1 inch of boiling water. Cover and steam the broccoli until fork-tender but still bright green and a little crunchy.

Enjoying Raw. Broccoli florets make great crudités for parties and are an easy snack.

Eating Out. Broccoli is common in restaurant kitchens, so I often have it when dining out. I usually ask for it steamed. At Italian restaurants, I might treat myself to broccoli rabe, which has smaller florets and tiny leaves. With garlic and just a little oil, it's delicious!

Growing. One summer I picked up a couple of starter broccoli plants at a local nursery and planted them along with the tomatoes. By midsummer, the plants had grown large, with little florets.

9. Watch out for lead. Although banned from house paint for decades, lead still makes its way into your home on the soles of your feet and in newsprint (burning newspapers can liberate it into the air), drinking water (charcoal filtration removes most of it), lead-soldered cans, and ceramic cookware. You can significantly decrease environmental exposure by taking the steps recommended here as well as regularly washing your hands and damp mopping all horizontal surfaces, including windowsills.

Summary of Chapter Nine: Detoxify—and Lose Weight

1. Environmental toxins can cause inflammation and slowing of your metabolism, especially if you have allergies or sensitivities.
2. Your body is continuously destroying and removing toxins. Most of this work is done by enzymes in your liver, kidneys, intestines, lungs, and skin. Detoxifying enzymes need nutrients to function well.
3. Most "detox" programs deplete your body of the vital nutrients needed for detoxification. Instead of strengthening your innate ability to detoxify, they weaken it.
4. The Fat Resistance Diet supplies an abundance of crucial detoxification nutrients, making it the only detox diet you should ever need.

PART THREE

Meal Plans and Recipes

Welcome to the meal plans and recipes that are the heart of the Fat Resistance Diet. Because we know that the only way to help people to stay on a diet is to make the food amazing, we have worked with gusto to bring you the best, healthiest dishes possible. In the pages that follow, you'll find updates of American classics that you can enjoy the healthy way, as well as some great new flavors from around the world. We want to give you recipes that are more like the recipes of Rachael Ray, Tyler Florence, or Jamie Oliver, and less like diet food. So each step of the way from shopping cart to kitchen table, we've kept your needs in mind. We know you want food that is quick, simple, and delicious. Most of all delicious. This is food that we ourselves want to eat, and that's why we are so thrilled to bring it to you.

The meal plans outline what you should eat each day: breakfast, lunch, dinner, dessert, and a morning and afternoon snack. It looks like a lot of food, and it is. The meal plans were designed to give you the maximum satisfaction and nutrition to enable you to lose weight. We want you to embrace a new way of eating and watch the pounds melt away.

Stage 1

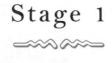

Meal Plan

Weeks 1 and 2

Stage 1 promotes rapid weight loss by aggressively targeting and reducing your inflammation. Abundant Fat Resistance Foods make this happen, which means nine to ten servings of fruits and vegetables a day, plus a generous amount of protein. This high level of nutrition will dramatically improve your body chemistry, lowering your insulin levels and allowing you to start shedding that stubborn extra weight. It is an especially good transition for people stuck on the very low-carb diets who can't get to a healthier diet because they gain weight as soon as they reintroduce more carbs. With Stage 1, sugar and starch cravings will disappear after two or three days, and by the end of this stage you will be on your way to successful long-term weight loss.

Day 1

On Arising
>   Slim Chai Tea

Breakfast
>   Tuscan Frittata
>   Fresh orange
>   Decaffeinated coffee with nonfat milk

Morning Snack
>   Blueberry Yogurt Cup
>   Slim Chai Tea

Lunch
>   Baby Spinach Salad with Apple and Roasted Walnuts
>   2 tablespoons Pomegranate Lime Dressing
>   Slim Chai Tea

Afternoon Snack
>   Vegetable juice
>   12 raw almonds

Dinner
>   Immune Power Soup
>   Green Tea–Crusted Salmon with Lemon Ginger Salsa
>   2 cups steamed broccoli

Dessert
>   Black Forest Banana Split

Day 2

On Arising
    Slim Chai Tea

Breakfast
    Smart Start Smoothie
    Decaffeinated coffee with nonfat milk

Morning Snack
    8 walnut halves
    Slim Chai Tea

Lunch
    Immune Power Soup
    Tuna Avocado Lettuce Wrap
    Slim Chai Tea

Afternoon Snack
    Vegetable juice

Dinner
    Grilled Sirloin with Garlic and Herbs
    2 cups steamed green beans
    Garden Salad
    1 tablespoon Pomegranate Lime Dressing

Dessert
    Cinnamon Lemon Poached Pear with Cherry Syrup

Day 3

On Arising
   Slim Chai Tea

Breakfast
   Smoked Salmon Frittata
   Fresh orange
   Decaffeinated coffee with nonfat milk

Morning Snack
   Carrot and celery sticks with 1 teaspoon almond butter
   Slim Chai Tea

Lunch
   Portobello Pizza con Ricotta
   2 cups arugula
   1 tablespoon Pesto Vinaigrette
   Slim Chai Tea

Afternoon Snack
   Iced Mocha Latte
   8 walnut halves

Dinner
   Pomegranate Chicken
   Asparagus with Red Bell Pepper and Garlic
   Garden Salad
   1 teaspoon each extra virgin olive oil and lemon juice

Dessert
   Blueberry Parfait

Day 4

On Arising
    Slim Chai Tea

Breakfast
    Parsley and Tomato Omelet
    Fresh grapefruit
    Decaffeinated coffee with nonfat milk

Morning Snack
    1 cup broccoli florets
    Slim Chai Tea

Lunch
    Greek Salad
    Slim Chai Tea

Afternoon Snack
    Blueberry Yogurt Cup

Dinner
    Immune Power Soup
    Walnut-Crusted Fish
    Asian Coleslaw

Dessert
    Fruit Kebabs with Pomegranate Glaze

Day 5

On Arising
  Slim Chai Tea

Breakfast
  2 hard-boiled eggs
  1 sliced tomato
  Fresh grapefruit
  Decaffeinated coffee with nonfat milk

Morning Snack
  8 walnut halves
  Slim Chai Tea

Lunch
  Immune Power Soup
  Thai Turkey Wrap
  Slim Chai Tea

Afternoon Snack
  Pomegranate juice
  12 raw almonds

Dinner
  Grilled Vegetables with Tofu
  2 cups mixed salad greens
  1 tablespoon Pesto Vinaigrette

Dessert
  Frosty Yogurt

Day 6

On Arising
Slim Chai Tea

Breakfast
Frittata with Fresh Herbs and Cheese
Fresh orange
Decaffeinated coffee with nonfat milk

Morning Snack
Blueberry Yogurt Cup
Slim Chai Tea

Lunch
Gazpacho
2 cups mixed salad greens
1 tablespoon Pesto Vinaigrette
Slim Chai Tea

Afternoon Snack
Pomegranate juice
12 raw almonds

Dinner
Immune Power Soup
Five Spice Chicken
Sesame Cabbage with Carrot, Parsley, and Basil

Dessert
Baked Apple with Cinnamon and Walnuts

Day 7

STAGE 1

On Arising
   Slim Chai Tea

Breakfast
   Your Favorite Omelet
   Fresh grapefruit
   Decaffeinated coffee with nonfat milk

Morning Snack
   1 cup broccoli florets
   Slim Chai Tea

Lunch
   Baby Spinach Salad with Apple and Roasted Walnuts
   2 tablespoons Pomegranate Lime Dressing
   Slim Chai Tea

Afternoon Snack
   Vegetable juice
   12 raw almonds

Dinner
   Herb-Crusted Fish
   Pomodori con Mozzarella (Tomatoes with Mozzarella)
   2 cups arugula
   1 tablespoon Pesto Vinaigrette

Dessert
   Strawberry Mango Granita

Day 8

On Arising
  Slim Chai Tea

Breakfast
  Smart Start Smoothie
  Fresh grapefruit
  Decaffeinated coffee with nonfat milk

Morning Snack
  12 raw almonds
  Slim Chai Tea

Lunch
  Mexican Salad
  2 cups mixed salad greens
  Slim Chai Tea

Afternoon Snack
  Pomegranate juice

Dinner
  Immune Power Soup
  Chicken Parmigiano
  Garden Salad
  1 tablespoon Pesto Vinaigrette

Dessert
  ½ cantaloupe

Day 9

On Arising
    Slim Chai Tea

Breakfast
    Mushroom Frittata
    Fresh orange
    Decaffeinated coffee with nonfat milk

Morning Snack
    Carrot and celery sticks with 1 teaspoon almond butter
    Slim Chai Tea

Lunch
    Immune Power Soup
    Cottage Cheese with Apple and Walnuts
    Slim Chai Tea

Afternoon Snack
    Vegetable juice
    12 raw almonds

Dinner
    Korean-Style Beef and Vegetables
    Garden Salad
    1 tablespoon Pomegranate Lime Dressing

Dessert
    Blueberry Parfait

Day 10

On Arising
   Slim Chai Tea

Breakfast
   Tuscan Frittata
   Fresh orange
   Decaffeinated coffee with nonfat milk

Morning Snack
   8 walnut halves
   Slim Chai Tea

Lunch
   Immune Power Soup
   Tuna Avocado Lettuce Wrap
   Slim Chai Tea

Afternoon Snack
   Pomegranate juice
   12 raw almonds

Dinner
   Big Vegetable Bowl
   1 sliced apple sprinkled with cinnamon

Dessert
   Frosty Yogurt

Day 11

On Arising
    Slim Chai Tea

Breakfast
    Frittata with Fresh Herbs and Cheese
    Fresh grapefruit
    Decaffeinated coffee with nonfat milk

Morning Snack
    8 walnut halves
    Slim Chai Tea

Lunch
    Gazpacho
    2 cups mixed salad greens
    1 tablespoon Pesto Vinaigrette
    Slim Chai Tea

Afternoon Snack
    Pomegranate juice
    12 raw almonds

Dinner
    Immune Power Soup
    Seared Scallops served over 2 cups arugula
    1 baked sweet potato

Dessert
    Black Forest Banana Split

Day 12

On Arising
   Slim Chai Tea

Breakfast
   Smart Start Smoothie
   Fresh grapefruit
   Decaffeinated coffee with nonfat milk

Morning Snack
   1 cup broccoli florets
   Slim Chai Tea

Lunch
   Smoked Salmon, Arugula, and Endive Salad
   2 tablespoons Pomegranate Lime Dressing
   Slim Chai Tea

Afternoon Snack
   Vegetable juice

Dinner
   Immune Power Soup
   Citrus Chicken Kebabs with Vegetables
   2 cups mixed salad greens
   1 tablespoon Pesto Vinaigrette

Dessert
   Cinnamon Lemon Poached Pear with Cherry Syrup

Day 13

On Arising
   Slim Chai Tea

Breakfast
   Crispy Tofu served over mixed salad greens
   Fresh orange
   Decaffeinated coffee with nonfat milk

Morning Snack
   Blueberry Yogurt Cup
   Slim Chai Tea

Lunch
   Greek Salad
   Slim Chai Tea

Afternoon Snack
   Vegetable juice
   12 raw almonds

Dinner
   Immune Power Soup
   Cilantro Shrimp with Pomegranate Salsa
   2 cups steamed broccoli
   Garden Salad
   1 teaspoon each extra virgin olive oil and lemon juice

Dessert
   Strawberry Mango Granita

Day 14

On Arising
   Slim Chai Tea

Breakfast
   Parsley and Tomato Omelet
   Fresh grapefruit
   Decaffeinated coffee with nonfat milk

Morning Snack
   8 walnut halves
   Slim Chai Tea

Lunch
   Immune Power Soup
   Thai Turkey Wrap
   Slim Chai Tea

Afternoon Snack
   Pomegranate juice
   12 raw almonds

Dinner
   Grilled Vegetables with Tofu
   2 cups mixed salad greens
   1 tablespoon Pesto Vinaigrette

Dessert
   Cherry Mint Parfait

Stage 1

~~~

Recipes

Breakfasts

TUSCAN FRITTATA

This frittata captures the classic flavors of Tuscany: tomato, basil, garlic, and olive oil. It's paired with arugula or spinach to fill you up on vegetables and keep you satisfied. Egg whites are an excellent source of protein and basil has powerful anti-inflammatory effects. Garlic is also anti-inflammatory and boosts the immune system. We cook frittatas the traditional way, using only a frying pan and not the oven.

   Olive oil spray
   1 garlic clove, minced
   3 egg whites, lightly beaten
   ½ tomato, diced
   2 tablespoons chopped fresh basil
   ¼ teaspoon salt
   Freshly ground black pepper
   2 cups arugula or baby spinach

Heat a small nonstick frying pan. Coat the pan with olive oil spray, add the garlic, and cook for 1 to 2 minutes over medium heat. Pour the egg whites over the garlic and spread the tomato and basil over the eggs. Season with salt and pepper. Cook for 4 minutes, or until the eggs are set. Flip the frittata over and cook for 2 minutes more. Serve over a bed of arugula. Serves 1.

NUTRITION PER SERVING: 87 Calories | 11 g Protein | 7 g Carbohydrates | 2 g Fat

SMART START SMOOTHIE

STAGE 1

Quick and easy to make, this smoothie is perfect for a morning on the run. Frozen blueberries work very well, allowing you to enjoy a simple summer pleasure any time of year. Blueberries contain more antioxidants than any other food. Yogurt has protein and calcium, and has been shown to aid weight loss. Flaxseeds are the richest plant source of anti-inflammatory omega-3s. Pour your smoothie into a travel mug and you have a refreshing breakfast treat to go.

    1 cup nonfat plain yogurt
    1 cup fresh or frozen blueberries
    1 tablespoon freshly ground flaxseeds
    1 tablespoon whey protein concentrate

Pour 2 tablespoons water into a blender. Add the yogurt and blueberries. Blend until the berries have turned the yogurt a deep rich blue. Add the ground flaxseeds and whey protein. Blend until smooth. Pour into a tall glass and enjoy! Serves 1.

NUTRITION PER SERVING: 332 Calories | 15 g Protein | 45 g Carbohydrates | 5 g Fat

Stage 1: Recipes   **195**

SMOKED SALMON FRITTATA

Smoked salmon and scallions are an incredible combination; the satisfying smokiness of the fish is perfectly offset by the freshness of the scallions. This frittata is high in protein and supplies omega-3s. Serve it with arugula, which has powerful phytonutrients.

2 ounces smoked salmon

Olive oil spray

3 egg whites, lightly beaten

2 stalks scallions, chopped

2 cups baby arugula or baby spinach

Freshly ground black pepper

Slice the salmon into small pieces. Heat a small nonstick frying pan over medium heat, coat it with olive oil spray, and pour in the egg whites. Spread the scallions and salmon over the eggs. Cook for 4 minutes, or until the eggs are set; then flip the frittata over and cook for 2 minutes more. Serve with arugula on the side. Smoked salmon tends to be salty, so you need season only with black pepper. Serves 1.

NUTRITION PER SERVING: 149 Calories | 21 g Protein | 6 g Carbohydrates | 4 g Fat

PARSLEY AND TOMATO OMELET

The vibrant green freshness of parsley makes this omelet high in phytonutrients and flavor. Parsley is a rich source of inflammation-fighting carotenoids. Tomato supplies lycopene, which may help prevent cancer. Garlic is anti-inflammatory and gives an appetite-satisfying depth of flavor.

Olive oil spray
1 garlic clove, minced
3 egg whites, lightly beaten
¼ teaspoon salt
Freshly ground black pepper
5 cherry or grape tomatoes, halved
¼ cup chopped fresh parsley
2 cups arugula or mixed salad greens

Heat a small nonstick frying pan. Coat the pan with olive oil spray, add the garlic, and cook for 1 to 2 minutes over medium heat. Pour the egg whites over the garlic and season with salt and pepper. Spread the tomato and parsley evenly over the eggs and cook for 4 minutes, or until the eggs are set. Fold one side of the omelet over the other to form a half circle and cook for 2 minutes more. Serve over a bed of arugula. Serves 1.

NUTRITION PER SERVING: 96 Calories | 12 g Protein | 9 g Carbohydrates | 2 g Fat

FRITTATA WITH FRESH HERBS AND CHEESE

STAGE 1

Indulge in a healthy pleasure with this fantastic frittata. Gooey melted cheese and green herbs make this a satisfying breakfast. The vibrant green herbs give you a sense of well-being and a fresh start to your day.

Olive oil spray
1 garlic clove, minced
3 egg whites, lightly beaten
¼ teaspoon salt
Freshly ground black pepper
2 tablespoons chopped fresh herbs: parsley, cilantro, sage, basil, or chives
2 ounces any low-fat cheese that melts nicely, such as mozzarella or Monterey Jack
1 tomato, sliced

Heat a small nonstick frying pan. Coat the pan with olive oil spray, add the garlic, and cook for 1 to 2 minutes over medium heat. Pour the egg whites over the garlic and season with salt and pepper. Spread the herbs and cheese evenly over the eggs and cook for 4 minutes, or until the eggs are set. Flip the frittata over and cook for 2 minutes more. Plate with tomato slices on the side. Serves 1.

NUTRITION PER SERVING: 175 Calories | 19 g Protein | 11 g Carbohydrates | 7 g Fat

YOUR FAVORITE OMELET

An easy and appetizing way to get vegetables into breakfast, this omelet is packed with high-quality protein and phytonutrients. Enjoy making your own favorite combination from the choices listed here, or from other fresh vegetables or herbs.

> Olive oil spray
> A handful of your favorite vegetables—choose two or three:
>> Fresh parsley, chopped (or other fresh or dried herbs)
>> Tomato, chopped
>> Scallions, chives, or leeks, finely chopped
>> Spinach, chopped
>> White button or shiitake mushrooms, finely chopped
>> Green, red, or yellow bell peppers, finely chopped
> 3 egg whites, lightly beaten
> ¼ teaspoon salt
> Freshly ground black pepper
> 2 cups mixed salad greens

Heat a small nonstick frying pan over medium heat and coat it with olive oil spray. When using hard vegetables such as leeks, mushrooms, or peppers, add them to the pan first and sauté over medium heat until tender, 3 to 5 minutes. Spread the egg whites evenly over the sautéed vegetables and cook for 4 minutes, or until the eggs are set, then fold one side over the other and cook for 2 minutes more. When using herbs and soft vegetables such as parsley and tomato, add the egg whites to the pan first, then spread the herbs and vegetables evenly over the egg whites. Cook for 4 minutes, or until the eggs are set, then fold one side over the other and cook for 2 minutes more. Season with salt and pepper. Have fun with it and don't worry about the shape. I serve the omelet whole or cut it into pieces right in the pan. It's about freshness and bright colors. Serve with mixed salad greens on the side. Serves 1.

NUTRITION PER SERVING: 96 Calories | 12 g Protein | 9 g Carbohydrates | 2 g Fat

MUSHROOM FRITTATA

Mushrooms and scallions give this frittata a rich, satisfying flavor. Shiitake mushrooms and scallions are valued for their immune-boosting properties.

Olive oil spray

⅓ cup thinly sliced shiitake or white button mushrooms

¼ cup chopped scallions

3 egg whites, lightly beaten

¼ teaspoon salt

Freshly ground black pepper

2 cups mixed salad greens

Heat a small nonstick frying pan. Coat the pan with olive oil spray, add the mushrooms and scallions, and cook for 3 to 4 minutes over medium heat. Pour the egg whites over the vegetables and season with salt and pepper. Cook for 4 minutes, or until the eggs are set. Flip the frittata over and cook for 2 minutes more. Serve the frittata over a bed of mixed salad greens. Serves 1.

NUTRITION PER SERVING: 112 Calories | 12 g Protein | 13 g Carbohydrates | 1 g Fat

CRISPY TOFU

This recipe is going to change your mind about tofu. The marinade of soy sauce and spices soaks great flavor into the tofu. Soy protein makes tofu an important addition to a healthy diet, and provides potential cancer-fighting isoflavones. If you were wondering how to cook with tofu, you now have a quick and tasty way to prepare this highly nutritious food.

7 ounces firm or extra-firm tofu

1 tablespoon low-sodium soy sauce

¼ teaspoon ground ginger

¼ teaspoon turmeric

1 teaspoon toasted sesame oil

2 tablespoons finely chopped scallions

½ cup frozen green peas

2 cups mixed salad greens

Freshly ground black pepper

¼ cup chopped fresh parsley, for garnish

Drain the tofu, rinse with cold water, then pat dry. Cut the tofu into 2-inch squares, ¼ inch thick. In a bowl large enough to hold the tofu, mix the soy sauce, ginger, and turmeric. Place the tofu in the bowl and gently coat it well with the marinade. Heat a nonstick frying pan, add the sesame oil, and place the tofu in the pan. Let the tofu brown on one side for 2 minutes over medium heat without turning. Then add the scallions and cook, turning occasionally, until the tofu is a nice golden brown.

While the tofu is cooking, bring a small amount of water to a boil in a pot. Add the peas and steam just until tender, about 4 minutes. Drain the peas and toss them with the tofu. Serve over mixed greens. Grind a little pepper over the top and garnish with fresh parsley. Serves 2.

NUTRITION PER SERVING: 171 Calories | 15 g Protein | 13 g Carbohydrates | 8 g Fat

Lunches

STAGE 1

BABY SPINACH SALAD WITH APPLE AND ROASTED WALNUTS

Spinach salad is a lunchtime classic. It looks and tastes great, and gives you lots of vegetable nutrition. Spinach is an excellent source of carotenoids, lutein, and zeaxanthin, important nutrients for maintaining healthy vision.

8 walnut halves
3 cups baby spinach
1 medium apple, peeled, cored, and sliced
1 hard-boiled egg
Pinch of salt
Freshly ground black pepper

Preheat the oven to 350°F. Spread the walnuts on a baking pan and bake, turning occasionally, for 4 to 5 minutes, or until lightly browned. Remove from the oven and let cool.

Place the spinach in a salad bowl or take-away container and spread the apple slices and walnuts over the spinach. Slice the egg in half and place it on top. Season with salt and pepper. Add dressing when you are ready to eat so the salad stays crisp. Serves 1.

TIMESAVING TIP: You can usually find a bag of washed baby spinach in the grocery store. The leaves are tender and the perfect size for salad.

NUTRITION PER SERVING: 264 Calories | 9 g Protein | 27 g Carbohydrates | 15 g Fat

TUNA AVOCADO LETTUCE WRAP

One 6-ounce can water-packed tuna, drained

2 stalks scallions, finely chopped

2 tablespoons chopped fresh parsley

1 teaspoon extra virgin olive oil

Juice of ½ lime

¼ teaspoon salt

Freshly ground black pepper

¼ avocado, peeled and sliced thin

1 tomato, sliced

3 large romaine lettuce leaves

In a bowl, mix the tuna, scallions, parsley, extra virgin olive oil, lime juice, salt, and black pepper. Put one-third of the tuna mixture, avocado, and tomato on each romaine leaf and fold into a wrap. Serves 1.

NUTRITION PER SERVING: 311 Calories | 46 g Protein | 13 g Carbohydrates | 9 g Fat

PORTOBELLO PIZZA CON RICOTTA

Melted mozzarella, rich portobello, creamy ricotta. This is a fun, fast way to enjoy the flavor and satisfaction of pizza, without the crust.

2 portobello mushrooms
¼ cup nonfat ricotta cheese
4 slices tomato or ¼ cup canned crushed tomatoes
2 garlic cloves, minced
6 tablespoons shredded low-fat mozzarella cheese
2 tablespoons chopped fresh basil
Pinch of salt
Freshly ground black pepper

Preheat the oven to 375°F. Clean the mushrooms and remove the stems. Place the mushrooms top down on a nonstick baking sheet, and spread 2 tablespoons of ricotta across each mushroom. Add the tomato and garlic, then top with the mozzarella and basil. Bake for 10 minutes, or until the cheese is slightly browned. Season with salt and pepper. Serves 1.

NUTRITION PER SERVING: 167 Calories | 13 g Protein | 17 g Carbohydrates | 5 g Fat

GREEK SALAD

Greek salad is a great way to enjoy lots of vegetables for lunch. Olives, feta cheese, and thyme give this salad a robust flavor to satisfy your appetite. If feta cheese is not available, substitute any low-fat cheese or a sprinkle of Parmesan.

2 cups chopped romaine lettuce
1 tomato, chopped
1 cucumber, chopped
½ red onion, diced
¼ cup pitted black olives
2 teaspoons extra virgin olive oil
Juice of ½ lemon
¼ cup crumbled feta cheese
1 tablespoon chopped fresh thyme or ¼ teaspoon dried thyme
¼ teaspoon salt

In a salad bowl or take-away container, toss the lettuce, tomato, cucumber, onion, and olives. In a cup, whisk together the extra virgin olive oil and lemon juice and pour over the salad when you are ready to eat. Spread the feta cheese over the top. Sprinkle with the thyme and salt. Serves 2.

NUTRITION PER SERVING: 209 Calories | 14 g Protein | 16 g Carbohydrates | 12 g Fat

THAI TURKEY WRAP

STAGE 1

Fresh herbs bring authentic Thai flavor and lots of antioxidants to this wrap. The lemongrass powder is a nice touch if you can find it in the supermarket or specialty market.

4 ounces sliced roast turkey

1 tomato, sliced

2 stalks scallions, thinly sliced lengthwise

3 tablespoons chopped fresh cilantro or mint

3 large romaine lettuce leaves

Shake of lemongrass powder (optional)

¼ teaspoon salt

Freshly ground black pepper

Put a third of the turkey, tomato, scallions, and cilantro on each romaine leaf. Sprinkle with lemongrass powder, salt, and pepper, then fold into a wrap. Serves 1.

NUTRITION PER SERVING: 293 Calories | 33 g Protein | 9 g Carbohydrates | 8 g Fat

GAZPACHO

Fast and easy to make right in your blender, gazpacho is about freshness and big flavors. Bursting with beautiful tomato color, gazpacho is rich in antioxidants, including lycopene. This recipe combines a nice vegetable crunchiness with a touch of satisfying spiciness.

1½ pounds tomatoes
1 cucumber, peeled
1 yellow or red bell pepper
1 red onion, diced
2 garlic cloves, chopped
½ cup chopped fresh parsley
1½ cups tomato juice or tomato-based vegetable juice
Juice of 1 lime
1 tablespoon extra virgin olive oil
¼ teaspoon salt
Freshly ground black pepper

Roughly chop the tomatoes, cucumber, pepper, and onion and toss them into a blender. Add the garlic and parsley, and blend until chunky. Pour half the mixture into a bowl. Add the tomato juice, lime juice, and extra virgin olive oil to the remaining vegetables in the blender and blend again until smooth. Combine both mixtures and season with salt and pepper. Serve hot or cold, depending on the season. Help yourself to a generous serving. Serves 2.

NUTRITION FOR A 2-CUP SERVING: 120 Calories | 4 g Protein | 20 g Carbohydrates
| 4 g Fat

MEXICAN SALAD

STAGE 1

Crunchy and colorful, this is a fun salad with great nutrition. Beans are a good source of protein and fiber, and are very high in antioxidants. Walnut oil gives you omega-3s, and cumin fights inflammation.

One 15-ounce can garbanzo beans (chickpeas)
One 15-ounce can black beans
2 tomatoes, diced
1 red or yellow bell pepper, diced
½ cup chopped scallions
½ cup chopped celery
¼ cup chopped fresh cilantro or parsley
2 garlic cloves, minced
¼ teaspoon cumin
½ teaspoon salt
Freshly ground black pepper
1 tablespoon walnut oil
Juice of 1 lime
2 cups mixed salad greens

Rinse the beans with cold water and drain. In a large bowl, toss the garbanzos, black beans, tomatoes, bell pepper, scallions, celery, cilantro, garlic, cumin, salt, and pepper. Dress the salad with the walnut oil and lime juice, and serve over mixed salad greens. Serves 4.

NUTRITION PER SERVING: 245 Calories | 12 g Protein | 39 g Carbohydrates | 5 g Fat

COTTAGE CHEESE WITH APPLE AND WALNUTS

This is a really fast recipe for lunch on the go. You get protein and calcium from cottage cheese, fiber and inflammation-fighting flavonoids from apple, and omega-3s from walnuts.

1 cup cored and sliced apple

1 tablespoon lemon juice

1 cup low-fat cottage cheese

¼ cup walnuts

Sprinkle of cinnamon

Lightly coat the apple slices with the lemon juice. In a bowl or take-away container, mix the cottage cheese and apple slices. Top with the walnuts and a sprinkle of cinnamon. Serves 1.

NUTRITION PER SERVING: 386 Calories | 32 g Protein | 26 g Carbohydrates | 19 g Fat

SMOKED SALMON, ARUGULA, AND ENDIVE SALAD

This bold salad rewards you with lots of flavor. Peppery arugula and crunchy endive perfectly complement the smokiness of the salmon.

  2 cups arugula or mixed salad greens
  1 head Belgian endive, chopped, or ½ cup chopped celery
  2 stalks scallions, chopped
  4 ounces smoked salmon, sliced
  1 teaspoon capers, rinsed
  Freshly ground black pepper
  1 teaspoon extra virgin olive oil
  1 teaspoon lime juice

In a bowl or take-away container, mix the arugula, endive, and scallions. Place the salmon slices on top of the salad, then add the capers and black pepper. Dress with the extra virgin olive oil and lime juice just before serving. Serves 1.

NUTRITION PER SERVING: 184 Calories | 23 g Protein | 11 g Carbohydrates | 5 g Fat

Dinners

GREEN TEA–CRUSTED SALMON WITH LEMON GINGER SALSA

This is a fantastic restaurant-style dish that you can make at home. The green tea rub gives the salmon a nice crunchy crust. Green tea is a great source of anti-inflammatory flavonoids. Salmon is also anti-inflammatory and provides omega-3 fatty acids.

Green Tea–Crusted Salmon

Olive oil spray

Two 8-ounce salmon fillets

2 tablespoons loose green tea

1 teaspoon sesame seeds

½ teaspoon garlic powder

½ teaspoon dried onion

Freshly ground black pepper

2 tablespoons low-sodium soy sauce

Lemon Ginger Salsa

2 tomatoes, chopped

1 apple, cored and diced

2 stalks scallions, finely chopped

Juice of 1 lemon

1 tablespoon peeled, minced fresh ginger

  or 1 teaspoon ground ginger

Preheat the oven to 400°F. Spray a pan with olive oil. Rinse the salmon with cold water and pat dry with a paper towel. In a shallow bowl, mix the green tea, sesame seeds, garlic powder, onion, and pepper. Pour the soy sauce into another shallow bowl, then dip the salmon in the soy sauce and coat well. Take the salmon out of the soy sauce and press it into the green tea rub, allowing the spices to stick to the top and sides of the salmon. Place the salmon in the pan and cook for 12 minutes, or until the center of the salmon turns from red to pink.

For the salsa, toss the tomatoes, apple, and scallions in a bowl, and sprinkle the lemon juice on top. Add the ginger and mix well. Place half the salsa next to each salmon portion. Serves 2.

NUTRITION PER SERVING: 292 Calories | 26 g Protein | 29 g Carbohydrates | 8 g Fat

GRILLED SIRLOIN WITH GARLIC AND HERBS

STAGE 1

Garlic and herbs have a robust flavor that work perfectly with grilled meat, and they're high in antioxidants. Cherry concentrate is packed with inflammation-fighting flavonoids. You can usually find cherry concentrate in a health food store with the bottled juices. Or see the Resources section in the back of the book for producers. Used as a marinade, cherry concentrate makes steak healthier because it reduces free radicals.

4 garlic cloves
2 tablespoons chopped fresh parsley
2 tablespoons low-sodium soy sauce
2 tablespoons cherry concentrate
1 tablespoon chopped fresh rosemary
1 tablespoon chopped fresh thyme leaves
Freshly ground black pepper
12 ounces sirloin steak
Olive oil spray

In a mini food processor, mince the garlic and parsley, then add the soy sauce and cherry concentrate and process until well combined. Pour the mixture into a shallow bowl and stir in the rosemary, thyme, and black pepper. Put the sirloin in the bowl and coat well with the marinade. Place the covered bowl in the refrigerator and let the sirloin marinate for 20 minutes.

Heat an electric grill or grill pan over medium-high heat. Spray the grill with olive oil. Place the sirloin on the grill and cook for 5 minutes on each side, or until medium. Remove from the grill and let the sirloin sit for 5 minutes, then slice. Serves 2.

NUTRITION PER SERVING: 391 Calories | 53 g Protein | 10 g Carbohydrates | 14 g Fat

POMEGRANATE CHICKEN

STAGE 1

Pomegranate juice is super high in antioxidants, and can usually be found refrigerated in your supermarket. You can also find where to buy pomegranate juice in the Resources section in the back of this book.

Two 8-ounce skinless, boneless chicken breasts
¼ cup unsweetened pomegranate juice
Juice of 1 lemon or lime
1 teaspoon extra virgin olive oil
2 garlic cloves, minced
½ cup chopped fresh parsley
¼ teaspoon salt
Freshly ground black pepper
Olive oil spray
3 cups chopped romaine lettuce

Cut the chicken into thin slices. To make the marinade, mix the pomegranate juice, lemon juice, extra virgin olive oil, garlic, and parsley in a large bowl. Season with salt and pepper. Add the chicken and coat well with the marinade. Cover the bowl and place in the refrigerator for 10 minutes to marinate.

Heat a nonstick frying pan and coat it with olive oil spray. Put the chicken in the pan and cook over medium heat for 7 to 8 minutes, turning occasionally, until cooked through. Discard the remaining marinade. Serve the chicken over a bed of romaine lettuce. Serves 2.

NUTRITION PER SERVING: 290 Calories | 54 g Protein | 9 g Carbohydrates | 4 g Fat

WALNUT-CRUSTED FISH

1 pound flounder, sole, or tilapia fillets

2 egg whites

1 cup finely chopped walnuts

¼ teaspoon salt

Freshly ground black pepper

Olive oil spray

Juice of ½ lemon

¼ cup finely chopped fresh parsley, for garnish

Rinse the fish in cold water and pat dry with a paper towel. Beat the egg whites in a shallow bowl. Spread the chopped walnuts, salt, and pepper on a plate. Dip the fish in the egg whites and then dredge in the walnut mixture, gently pressing the walnuts onto the fish to form the crust.

Heat a nonstick skillet and coat it with olive oil spray. Place the fish in the skillet and cook over medium heat for 3 to 4 minutes each side, until the fish is cooked through. Squeeze lemon juice over the top, then sprinkle with parsley. Serves 2.

NUTRITION PER SERVING: 427 Calories | 49 g Protein | 6 g Carbohydrates | 24 g Fat

GRILLED VEGETABLES WITH TOFU

This is a fantastic way to eat vegetables. You get great grilled flavor using a grill pan or electric grill, and the result is vegetables that are chewy, filling, and satisfying. Tofu adds protein, making this a complete meal.

    One 14-ounce package firm or extra-firm tofu
    Six ½-inch-thick slices eggplant
    6 mushrooms, sliced
    1 red, yellow, or green bell pepper, thinly sliced
    4 plum tomatoes, halved
    2 garlic cloves, halved
    ½ onion, sliced
    Olive oil spray
    ¼ teaspoon salt
    Freshly ground black pepper
    ¼ cup chopped fresh parsley, for garnish

Heat an electric grill or grill pan. Cut the tofu into ¼-inch-thick slices. Mist the eggplant, mushrooms, bell pepper, tomatoes, garlic, onion, and tofu with olive oil spray, sprinkle with salt and pepper, then put on the grill. (You may do this in batches.) Cook for 2 to 3 minutes on each side over medium-high heat, until the vegetables are a little tender and the tofu is browned. Remove from the grill and shower with fresh parsley. Serves 2.

NUTRITION PER SERVING: 328 Calories | 27 g Protein | 38 g Carbohydrates | 10 g Fat

FIVE SPICE CHICKEN

1 tablespoon low-sodium soy sauce

1 tablespoon toasted sesame oil

½ cup chopped scallions

1 teaspoon peeled, finely chopped fresh ginger

2 garlic cloves, minced

½ teaspoon five-spice powder

¼ teaspoon turmeric

1 pound skinless, boneless chicken breasts, cut into strips

Olive oil spray

4 cups chopped romaine lettuce

2 tablespoons chopped fresh cilantro, for garnish

To make the marinade, whisk together the soy sauce, sesame oil, scallions, ginger, garlic, five-spice powder, and turmeric in a large bowl. Add the chicken and coat well with the mixture, then marinate, covered, in the refrigerator for 10 minutes.

Heat a nonstick frying pan and coat with olive oil spray. Add the chicken strips and cook over medium heat for 5 to 6 minutes, turning once or twice, until cooked through. Place on a bed of romaine lettuce and sprinkle with cilantro. Serves 2.

NUTRITION PER SERVING: 279 Calories | 53 g Protein | 5 g Carbohydrates | 4 g Fat

HERB-CRUSTED FISH

Fresh herbs give this dish its satisfying flavor and vibrant green color. It's quick and easy to make using a handful of fresh herbs from the garden or supermarket. Herbs are a rich source of phytonutrients and antioxidants.

1 pound flounder, sole, or tilapia fillets

2 egg whites

¼ cup chopped fresh herbs: parsley, basil, rosemary, sage, or dill

2 garlic cloves, minced

¼ teaspoon salt

Freshly ground black pepper

Olive oil spray

Juice of ½ lemon

Rinse the fish fillets in cold water and pat dry with a paper towel. Beat the egg whites in a shallow bowl. Spread the herbs, garlic, salt, and pepper on a plate. Dip the fillets in the egg whites, then dredge them in the herb mixture, pressing the herbs onto the fish.

Heat a nonstick skillet. Coat the skillet with olive oil spray, then add the fillets. Cook over medium heat for 3 to 4 minutes on each side, until the fish is cooked through. Plate the fish and finish with a squeeze of lemon. Serves 2.

NUTRITION PER SERVING: 295 Calories | 59 g Protein | 3 g Carbohydrates | 4 g Fat

CHICKEN PARMIGIANO

This is a healthy update on a classic. Red tomatoes, melted mozzarella, and green basil are all here. Plus it's so easy to make, you will be delighted at how quickly you can prepare this great-looking dish.

1 pound skinless, boneless chicken breasts
Olive oil spray
1½ cups canned crushed tomatoes
3 tablespoons low-fat ricotta cheese
¼ teaspoon salt
Freshly ground black pepper
2 garlic cloves, minced
1 cup shredded low-fat mozzarella cheese
¼ cup chopped fresh basil

Preheat the oven to 375°F. Rinse the chicken with cold water and pat dry with a paper towel. Spray a nonstick baking pan with olive oil. Arrange the breasts on the pan, then cover with the tomatoes and ricotta. Season with salt and pepper and sprinkle with the garlic, mozzarella, and basil. Bake for 35 minutes, or until the chicken is cooked through, the ricotta is bubbling hot, and the mozzarella turns golden brown. Serves 2.

NUTRITION PER SERVING: 379 Calories | 74 g Protein | 10 g Carbohydrates | 3 g Fat

KOREAN-STYLE BEEF AND VEGETABLES

STAGE

This is a tastier and healthier way to eat beef because the marinade is made with pomegranate juice. Cabbage, bok choy, and napa cabbage are excellent sources of cancer-fighting nutrients, and garlic reduces inflammation.

3 tablespoons low-sodium soy sauce

1 tablespoon toasted sesame oil

¼ cup finely chopped scallions

3 garlic cloves, minced

2 tablespoons unsweetened pomegranate juice

8 ounces stir-fry beef or flank steak

4 cups chopped bok choy, Napa cabbage, or green cabbage

3 cups chopped romaine lettuce

1 teaspoon sesame seeds, for garnish

To make the marinade, whisk together the soy sauce and sesame oil in a bowl large enough to hold the beef. Add the scallions, garlic, and pomegranate juice and mix well. Slice the beef into ½-inch strips and put in the bowl, coating the beef well with the marinade. Cover the bowl and place in the refrigerator to marinate for 15 minutes.

Heat a nonstick frying pan. Place the strips of beef in the pan and cook over medium heat for 2 to 3 minutes, until the meat is done. Discard the marinade. Transfer the meat to a bowl. Put the bok choy in the heated pan and stir-fry over medium-high heat for 4 minutes. Return the cooked beef to the pan and mix with the bok choy, then remove from the heat.

To serve, put the beef and bok choy on a bed of romaine lettuce. Sprinkle with sesame seeds. Serves 2.

NUTRITION PER SERVING: 233 Calories | 23 g Protein | 15 g Carbohydrates | 9 g Fat

BIG VEGETABLE BOWL

Big. Crunchy. Satisfying. This dish overflows with nourishing vegetables. Quickly sautéed, the vegetables stay crisp and delicious. You get lots of inflammation-fighting flavonoids, plus fiber, vitamins, and minerals. Tofu adds protein and makes this a complete meal.

Olive oil spray

4 garlic cloves, chopped

½ cup chopped onion

1 tablespoon peeled, minced fresh ginger

One 14-ounce package firm or extra-firm tofu

2 carrots, sliced into thin rounds

1 cup sliced white button or shiitake mushrooms

2 cups broccoli florets

¼ teaspoon turmeric

¼ teaspoon salt

Freshly ground black pepper

4 cups baby spinach or one 10-ounce package frozen spinach, thawed
   and squeezed dry

1 tablespoon low-sodium soy sauce

1 teaspoon sesame seeds, for garnish

Heat a nonstick frying pan, then coat with olive oil spray. Cook the garlic, onion, and ginger over medium heat for 3 to 4 minutes, stirring occasionally. Drain the tofu, pat it dry, and cut it into 1-inch cubes. Add the tofu, carrots, mushrooms, and broccoli to the pan; season with turmeric, salt, and pepper; then cook for 5 minutes over medium heat. Add the spinach and cook for 3 to 4 minutes more, until the spinach wilts. Place the vegetables in a large bowl and sprinkle with soy sauce and sesame seeds. Serves 2.

NUTRITION PER SERVING: 357 Calories | 32 g Protein | 33 g Carbohydrates | 14 g Fat

SEARED SCALLOPS

1 pound sea scallops

Juice of 1 lemon or lime

2 garlic cloves, sliced

Pinch of salt

Freshly ground black pepper

Olive oil spray

2 tablespoons chopped fresh parsley

Rinse the scallops and pat dry with a paper towel. Mix the lemon juice, garlic, salt, and pepper in a shallow bowl. Add the scallops and toss to coat well, then marinate, covered, in the refrigerator for 10 minutes.

Heat a nonstick frying pan and coat with olive oil spray. Using a slotted spoon, transfer the scallops and garlic to the pan. Cook over medium-high heat for 3 to 4 minutes, until the scallops are nicely browned. Turn the scallops over and sprinkle with parsley. Cook for 2 minutes more, or until the scallops are firm. Serves 3.

NUTRITION PER SERVING: 144 Calories | 25 g Protein | 6 g Carbohydrates | 2 g Fat

CITRUS CHICKEN KEBABS WITH VEGETABLES

Citrus and parsley give this dish a wonderful freshness. Grilling the chicken with vegetables and lemon wedges imparts a lot of flavor to the kebabs.

Two 8-ounce skinless, boneless chicken breasts
1 tablespoon extra virgin olive oil
Juice of 1 lemon
¼ teaspoon salt
Freshly ground black pepper
¼ cup finely chopped parsley
6 white button mushrooms, halved if large
8 cherry or grape tomatoes
½ onion, cut into 4 wedges
2 lemons, cut into wedges

Cut the chicken into 1-inch cubes. To make the marinade, whisk together the extra virgin olive oil, lemon juice, salt, and pepper, then mix in the chopped parsley. Marinate the chicken, covered, in the refrigerator for 10 minutes. Remove the chicken from the marinade and thread onto metal skewers, alternating with the mushrooms, tomatoes, and onion and lemon wedges. Discard the remaining marinade. (If you use wooden skewers, soak them in cold water for at least an hour before using to prevent them from burning.)

Heat an electric grill or grill pan. Place the skewers on the grill and cook for 5 to 6 minutes, turning occasionally, until the chicken is cooked through. Remove the chicken and vegetables from the skewers. Serves 2.

NUTRITION PER SERVING: 310 Calories | 25 g Protein | 14 g Carbohydrates | 18 g Fat

CILANTRO SHRIMP
WITH POMEGRANATE SALSA

The bright citrus flavor of lime and vibrant freshness of cilantro work perfectly with shrimp. The salsa adds a touch of sweetness to these big flavors.

Cilantro Shrimp

Juice of 1 lime

1 tablespoon extra virgin olive oil

½ cup chopped fresh cilantro

Freshly ground black pepper

½ pound large shrimp, peeled and deveined

Pomegranate Salsa

1 cup chopped tomatoes

¼ cup diced sweet onion

¼ cup finely chopped yellow bell pepper

Juice of ½ lime

2 tablespoons unsweetened pomegranate juice

To marinate the shrimp, put the lime juice, extra virgin olive oil, cilantro, and black pepper in a blender and puree. Pour the mixture into a large bowl and add the cleaned shrimp, coating the shrimp well. Cover the bowl and refrigerate for 30 minutes.

While the shrimp are marinating, prepare the salsa. Combine the tomatoes, onion, and yellow pepper in a bowl. Add the lime juice and pomegranate juice and mix well.

Preheat the broiler. Place the marinated shrimp on a rimmed baking sheet and broil for 5 minutes, turning once. Discard the marinade. Serve the salsa with the shrimp. Serves 2.

NUTRITION PER SERVING: 176 Calories | 25 g Protein | 16 g Carbohydrates | 4 g Fat

SLIM CHAI TEA

2 green tea bags
10 whole cloves
¼ teaspoon cinnamon
¼ teaspoon cardamom

Bring 3 cups water to a boil. Remove from the heat, add the tea bags and cloves, and let steep for 3 minutes. Remove the tea bags and cloves. Add the cinnamon and cardamom and mix well. Serves 3.

BLUEBERRY YOGURT CUP

According to research, blueberries may have powerful anti-aging effects. The more the berrier. Enjoy!

½ cup fresh or frozen blueberries, thawed
1 cup nonfat plain yogurt

In a small bowl or take-away container, gently mix the blueberries into the yogurt. Serves 1.

NUTRITION PER SERVING: 141 Calories | 10 g Protein | 30 g Carbohydrates | 0.2 g Fat

ICED MOCHA LATTE

Rich and creamy, this latte has a robust chocolate and coffee flavor that is very satisfying. This is going to become one of your favorite drinks.

 1½ cups nonfat milk or unsweetened soymilk
 1 teaspoon unsweetened cocoa powder
 1 teaspoon instant coffee

In a blender, combine the milk, cocoa powder, and instant coffee and blend until foamy. Pour into a tall glass with ice. Serves 1.

WITH NONFAT MILK NUTRITION PER SERVING: 134 Calories | 13 g Protein |
19 g Carbohydrates | 1 g Fat

WITH SOYMILK NUTRITION PER SERVING: 156 Calories | 11 g Protein |
13 g Carbohydrates | 6 g Fat

Soups, Sides, and Dressings

POMEGRANATE LIME DRESSING

STAGE

Pomegranate juice is an outstanding source of flavonoids, which help to reduce inflammation.

> 1 teaspoon extra virgin olive oil or walnut oil
> Juice of ½ lime
> 1 tablespoon unsweetened pomegranate juice

In a jar, shake together the extra virgin olive oil, lime juice, and pomegranate juice. Serves 1.

NUTRITION PER SERVING: 66 Calories | 0.17 g Protein | 7 g Carbohydrates | 5 g Fat

IMMUNE POWER SOUP

STAGE

This soup takes the edge off your hunger and is a great way to get more vegetables into your day. Make it in advance and freeze it in single-serving containers for use later on.

1 tablespoon extra virgin olive oil
2 cups sliced carrots
1 cup chopped leeks, white and light green parts only, rinsed thoroughly
1 cup chopped celery
1 cup diced onions
4 garlic cloves, minced
1 tablespoon peeled, minced fresh ginger
1 cup finely sliced shiitake mushrooms
1 cup chopped fresh parsley
¼ cup chopped fresh basil
1 teaspoon salt
Freshly ground black pepper
¼ cup chopped fresh chives, for garnish

Heat the extra virgin olive oil in a large pot. Add the carrots, leeks, celery, onions, garlic, and ginger and sauté for 10 minutes over medium heat, stirring frequently.

Add the shiitake mushrooms, parsley, basil, and 8 cups water. Season with salt and pepper. Turn the heat to high and bring to a boil; then reduce the heat to medium-low and simmer, covered, for 20 minutes. Serve in a bowl or mug and garnish with chives. Serves 5.

NUTRITION PER SERVING: 90 Calories | 2 g Protein | 14 g Carbohydrates | 3 g Fat

GARDEN SALAD

2 cups mixed salad greens

4 cherry or grape tomatoes, halved

4 slices cucumber

4 slices red, yellow, or green bell pepper

In a bowl, toss the greens, tomatoes, cucumber, and pepper. Serves 1.

NUTRITION PER SERVING: 37 Calories | 3 g Protein | 7 g Carbohydrates | 0.5 g Fat

PESTO VINAIGRETTE

1 cup fresh basil leaves

2 tablespoons extra virgin olive oil

1 tablespoon vinegar

1 garlic clove

Pinch of salt

Freshly ground black pepper

Put the basil in a mini food processor, pour in the extra virgin olive oil, and blend. Add the vinegar, garlic, salt, and pepper and blend until smooth. Serves 2.

NUTRITION PER SERVING: 63 Calories | 0.25 g Protein | 3 g Carbohydrates | 6 g Fat

ASPARAGUS WITH RED BELL PEPPER AND GARLIC

Add a splash of color and flavor to your asparagus with diced red bell pepper and garlic.

12 stalks asparagus, peeled, trimmed, and washed
Olive oil spray
2 garlic cloves, minced
½ red bell pepper, finely diced
Juice of ½ lemon
Pinch of salt
Freshly ground black pepper

Soak the asparagus in warm water for 10 minutes and rinse. Bring an inch or two of water to a boil in a skillet or pot large enough to hold the asparagus. Place the asparagus in the steamer or on a steaming rack in the skillet and steam until fork-tender, about 5 minutes. While the asparagus is cooking, heat a frying pan and coat it with olive oil spray. Add the garlic and bell pepper and cook for 4 minutes over medium heat. If the garlic starts to brown, lower the heat.

Drain the asparagus and toss with the garlic and pepper. Finish with the lemon juice and season with salt and black pepper. Serves 2.

NUTRITION PER SERVING: 56 Calories | 4 g Protein | 11 g Carbohydrates | 0.87 g Fat

ASIAN COLESLAW

Crunchy, tangy, and just a little spicy, this is the healthy way to enjoy coleslaw.

STAGE

4 cups shredded green cabbage

½ cup finely sliced onion

½ cup finely sliced carrot

Juice of ½ lime

2 teaspoons low-sodium soy sauce

2 teaspoons toasted sesame oil

¼ teaspoon salt

¼ teaspoon freshly ground black pepper

In a large bowl, combine the cabbage, onion, and carrot. In a small bowl, whisk together the lime juice, soy sauce, sesame oil, salt, and pepper. When ready to serve, pour the dressing over the vegetables and mix well. Serves 4.

NUTRITION PER SERVING: 66 Calories | 2 g Protein | 11 g Carbohydrates | 2 g Fat

SESAME CABBAGE WITH CARROT, PARSLEY, AND BASIL

1 teaspoon toasted sesame oil

4 cups shredded green cabbage

1 cup finely sliced onions

1 cup julienned carrots

¼ teaspoon salt

¼ teaspoon freshly ground black pepper

½ cup chopped fresh parsley

¼ cup chopped fresh basil

Heat a nonstick skillet large enough to hold the vegetables, and add the sesame oil. Add the cabbage, onions, carrots, salt, and pepper and cook over medium heat for 5 to 6 minutes, stirring frequently, until the vegetables become slightly tender. Mix in the parsley and basil and cook for 1 minute more. Serves 2.

NUTRITION PER SERVING: 112 Calories | 4 g Protein | 21 g Carbohydrates | 3 g Fat

POMODORI CON MOZZARELLA
Tomatoes with Mozzarella

This dish will make you feel as if you are eating in a restaurant. It looks fantastic and is very easy to make. Ripe tomatoes, melted mozzarella, garlic, and a sprinkle of parsley make this a rich and satisfying side dish.

Olive oil spray
4 slices tomato
Pinch of salt
2 garlic cloves, minced
2 tablespoons shredded low-fat mozzarella cheese
2 teaspoons grated Parmesan cheese
2 tablespoons finely chopped fresh parsley, for garnish

Preheat the broiler in your oven or toaster oven. Spray a nonstick baking pan with olive oil and place the tomato slices on the pan. Sprinkle salt on the tomatoes, then broil for 4 minutes. Remove the tomatoes from the oven and spread them with the garlic, mozzarella, and Parmesan. Broil again for 5 minutes, or until the cheese is golden brown. Sprinkle the parsley over the melted cheese. Serves 2.

NUTRITION PER SERVING: 38 Calories | 3 g Protein | 3 g Carbohydrates | 2 g Fat

Desserts

BLACK FOREST BANANA SPLIT

1 cup nonfat ricotta cheese

1 banana, split lengthwise

8 walnut halves

½ teaspoon unsweetened cocoa powder

1 teaspoon cherry concentrate

Spoon the ricotta into a dessert dish and place a banana half on each side of the cheese. Put the walnut halves on top and dust with the cocoa powder. Drizzle the cherry concentrate on top. Serves 1.

NUTRITION PER SERVING: 377 Calories | 23 g Protein | 40 g Carbohydrates | 11 g Fat

CINNAMON LEMON POACHED PEARS WITH CHERRY SYRUP

This is a delightful fruit dessert with layers of flavor and lots of antioxidants.

- 2 ripe pears
- 1 tablespoon cherry concentrate
- Juice of ½ lemon
- 1 teaspoon cinnamon
- 2 tablespoons chopped raw almonds
- 2 mint sprigs, for garnish

Peel and core the pears. Combine the pears, 1 cup water, the cherry concentrate, lemon juice, and cinnamon in a saucepan. Cover and simmer for 7 to 10 minutes, until fork-tender. With a slotted spoon, transfer the pears to two shallow bowls. Simmer the liquid until it is reduced to a syrup and spoon over the pears. Top with the chopped almonds and mint. Serves 2.

NUTRITION PER SERVING: 177 Calories | 3 g Protein | 33 g Carbohydrates | 6 g Fat

BLUEBERRY PARFAIT

Blueberry concentrate gives this dessert a deep hue and is rich in flavonoids. See the Resources section in the back of this book for sources or try your local health food store.

1 cup nonfat plain yogurt
½ cup fresh or frozen blueberries, thawed
1 teaspoon blueberry concentrate

In a parfait or wine glass, layer the yogurt, blueberries, and blueberry concentrate. Serves 1.

NUTRITION PER SERVING: 156 Calories | 11 g Protein | 30 g Carbohydrates | 0.24 g Fat

FRUIT KEBABS WITH POMEGRANATE GLAZE

Juice of ½ lemon
2 tablespoons unsweetened pomegranate juice
1 banana, thickly sliced
6 strawberries
6 pineapple chunks

Preheat the oven to 350°F. Combine the lemon juice and pomegranate juice in a bowl large enough to hold the fruit. Add the banana, strawberries, and pineapple and coat well with the mixture. Thread the fruit onto skewers, set the skewers on a nonstick baking pan, and bake for 7 to 8 minutes, until the fruit is bubbly. Serves 2.

NUTRITION PER SERVING: 226 Calories | 3 g Protein | 59 g Carbohydrates | 0.83 g Fat

FROSTY YOGURT

The goodness of berries shines through in this healthy treat. It's a snap to make and can be prepared in advance.

    1 cup frozen blueberries, strawberries, or mixed berries
    1 cup nonfat plain yogurt

Toss the frozen berries into a blender and add 2 tablespoons water. Blend until the berries are well chopped. Add the yogurt and blend until smooth. Spoon into bowls and enjoy, or store in an airtight container in the freezer. Serves 2.

NUTRITION PER SERVING: 90 Calories | 5 g Protein | 19 g Carbohydrates | 0.5 g Fat

BAKED APPLES WITH CINNAMON AND WALNUTS

Imagine walking into a kitchen filled with the rich aroma of cinnamon and apples baking in the oven. This is comfort food at its best. The sweetness of soft, warm apples is enhanced by pomegranate syrup, and the walnuts are crunchy and satisfying.

    2 apples for baking, such as McIntosh, cored
    1 cup unsweetened pomegranate juice
    1 teaspoon cinnamon
    16 walnut halves

Preheat the oven to 350°F. Place the apples in a baking dish. Pour the pomegranate juice over the apples. This will become a syrup as the apples cook. Sprinkle with the cinnamon and bake for 30 minutes, basting with the syrup, or until the apples are soft, but still hold their shape. Serve each apple topped with walnuts and syrup. Serves 2.

NUTRITION PER SERVING: 251 Calories | 3 g Protein | 41 g Carbohydrates | 11 g Fat

STRAWBERRY MANGO GRANITA

This fruit ice is pure pleasure with the sweetness of mango and the refreshing tartness of strawberries.

1 cup chopped mango
1 cup strawberries
1 cup crushed Ice

Puree the mango and strawberries in a blender. Add the ice and 5 tablespoons water and blend until smooth. Add a little more water if needed to mix well. Serve immediately or store in the freezer. (Before serving, remove from the freezer and let thaw until soft enough to break up with a fork.) Serves 2.

NUTRITION PER SERVING: 38 Calories | 1 g Protein | 9 g Carbohydrates | 0.33 g Fat

CHERRY MINT PARFAIT

1 cup nonfat plain yogurt
½ cup pitted fresh cherries
1 teaspoon cherry concentrate
4 fresh mint leaves, sliced

In a parfait or wine glass, layer the yogurt, cherries, and cherry concentrate. Top with the mint. Serves 1.

NUTRITION PER SERVING: 162 Calories | 11 g Protein | 35 g Carbohydrates | 0.15 g Fat

Stage 2

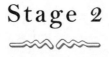

Meal Plan

Weeks 3, 4, and beyond

Stage 2 expands the range of Fat Resistance Foods choices, making it ideal for long-term weight loss. The meal plan is designed to allow you to comfortably lose two pounds per week, and to continue with this plan until you have reached your target weight. After completing Stage 1, you introduce grains such as oatmeal and brown rice, and increase the use of beans, to add fiber. What does all this mean for you? Now you get to enjoy lots of new recipes, such as Omega Blast Granola, Ginger Lime Grilled Tuna, and Pineapple Orange Granita, while you continue moderate weight loss. Sound good? That's the idea. Because we want you to stick with the plan until you reach your weight-loss goals.

Day 1

STAGE 2

On Arising
   Slim Chai Tea

Breakfast
   Omega Blast Granola with 1 cup nonfat plain yogurt,
      nonfat milk, or unsweetened soymilk and ½ apple,
      chopped
   Decaffeinated coffee with nonfat milk

Morning Snack
   Carrot and celery sticks
   Slim Chai Tea

Lunch
   Smoked Salmon, Arugula, and Endive Salad
   2 tablespoons Ginger Orange Dressing
   Slim Chai Tea

Afternoon Snack
   Vegetable juice

Dinner
   Immune Power Soup
   Apricot Mint Chicken
   ½ cup brown rice

Dessert
   1 cup fresh strawberries

Day 2

On Arising
   Slim Chai Tea

Breakfast
   Frittata with Tomato, Capers, and Cilantro
   Fresh grapefruit
   Decaffeinated coffee with nonfat milk

Morning Snack
   1 cup broccoli florets
   Slim Chai Tea

Lunch
   Immune Power Soup
   Basmati Rice Salad
   Slim Chai Tea

Afternoon Snack
   Iced Mocha Latte
   12 raw almonds

Dinner
   Ginger Lime Grilled Tuna
   Asian Coleslaw

Dessert
   Pineapple Orange Granita

Day 3

STAGE 2

On Arising
   Slim Chai Tea

Breakfast
   Blueberry Cinnamon Bowl
   Fresh grapefruit
   Decaffeinated coffee with nonfat milk

Morning Snack
   1 red or yellow bell pepper, sliced
   Slim Chai Tea

Lunch
   Immune Power Soup
   Insalata Caprese (Mozzarella and Tomato Salad)
   Slim Chai Tea

Afternoon Snack
   Pomegranate juice

Dinner
   Grilled Steak with Chimichurri Sauce
   Zucchini with Garlic and Herbs
   2 cups mixed salad greens

Dessert
   Cinnamon Lemon Poached Pear with Cherry Syrup

Day 4

On Arising
   Slim Chai Tea

Breakfast
   Banana Strawberry Smoothie
   Fresh grapefruit
   Decaffeinated coffee with nonfat milk

Morning Snack
   Carrot and celery sticks with 1 teaspoon almond butter
   Slim Chai Tea

Lunch
   Immune Power Soup
   Tofu "Egg" Salad
   Slim Chai Tea

Afternoon Snack
   Vegetable juice
   8 walnut halves

Dinner
   Ginger Infused Salmon
   Sesame Cabbage with Carrot, Parsley, and Basil

Dessert
   Fruit Kebabs with Pomegranate Glaze

Day 5

STAGE 2

On Arising
Slim Chai Tea

Breakfast
Smoked Salmon Frittata
Fresh orange
Decaffeinated coffee with nonfat milk

Morning Snack
8 walnut halves
Slim Chai Tea

Lunch
Summer Cool Cucumber Soup or
Winter Warm Tomato Basil Soup
Tuna Avocado Lettuce Wrap
Slim Chai Tea

Afternoon Snack
Pomegranate juice

Dinner
Immune Power Soup
Chicken Parmigiano
2 cups arugula
1 tablespoon Pesto Vinaigrette

Dessert
Frosty Yogurt

Day 6

On Arising
  Slim Chai Tea

Breakfast
  2 hard-boiled eggs
  1 tomato, sliced
  Fresh grapefruit
  Decaffeinated coffee with nonfat milk

Morning Snack
  Blueberry Yogurt Cup
  Slim Chai Tea

Lunch
  Portobello Pizza con Ricotta
  2 cups mixed salad greens
  1 tablespoon Lemon Spice Dressing
  Slim Chai Tea

Afternoon Snack
  Vegetable juice
  12 raw almonds

Dinner
  Immune Power Soup
  Roasted Salmon with Ginger, Garlic, and Scallions
  Sesame Cabbage with Carrot, Parsley, and Basil

Dessert
  Warm Spiced Apricots and Figs

Day 7

On Arising
   Slim Chai Tea

Breakfast
   Mushroom Frittata
   Fresh orange
   Decaffeinated coffee with nonfat milk

Morning Snack
   8 walnut halves
   Slim Chai Tea

Lunch
   Insalata Fagioli (Italian Bean Salad)
   Slim Chai Tea

Afternoon Snack
   Pomegranate juice
   12 raw almonds

Dinner
   Immune Power Soup
   Citrus Chicken Kebabs with Vegetables
   2 cups mixed salad greens
   1 tablespoon Pesto Vinaigrette

Dessert
   Blueberry Parfait

Day 8

On Arising
    Slim Chai Tea

Breakfast
    Omega Blast Granola with 1 cup nonfat plain yogurt,
        nonfat milk, or unsweetened soymilk and ½ apple,
        chopped
    Decaffeinated coffee with nonfat milk

Morning Snack
    Carrot and celery sticks
    Slim Chai Tea

Lunch
    Chicken Caesar Salad
    Slim Chai Tea

Afternoon Snack
    Pomegranate juice

Dinner
    Stir-Fried Vegetables with Beef or Tofu
    Asian Coleslaw

Dessert
    1 cup fresh strawberries

Day 9

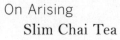

On Arising
  Slim Chai Tea

Breakfast
  Tuscan Frittata
  Fresh grapefruit
  Decaffeinated coffee with nonfat milk

Morning Snack
  8 walnut halves
  Slim Chai Tea

Lunch
  Immune Power Soup
  Asian Grilled Chicken Salad
  2 tablespoons Pomegranate Lime Dressing
  Slim Chai Tea

Afternoon Snack
  Iced Mocha Latte
  12 raw almonds

Dinner
  Herb-Crusted Fish
  Asparagus with Red Bell Pepper and Garlic
  Eggplant Tart

Dessert
  Cherry Mint Parfait

Day 10

On Arising
  Slim Chai Tea

Breakfast
  Smart Start Smoothie
  Fresh grapefruit
  Decaffeinated coffee with nonfat milk

Morning Snack
  1 cup broccoli florets
  Slim Chai Tea

Lunch
  Insalata Caprese (Mozzarella and Tomato Salad)
  Slim Chai Tea

Afternoon Snack
  Vegetable juice
  12 raw almonds

Dinner
  Teriyaki Chicken
  2 cups steamed green beans with lemon juice

Dessert
  Black Forest Banana Split

Day 11

STAGE 2

On Arising
   Slim Chai Tea

Breakfast
   Your Favorite Omelet
   Fresh orange
   Decaffeinated coffee with nonfat milk

Morning Snack
   8 walnut halves
   Slim Chai Tea

Lunch
   Mexican Salad
   Slim Chai Tea

Afternoon Snack
   Pomegranate juice
   12 raw almonds

Dinner
   Immune Power Soup
   Grilled Sirloin with Garlic and Herbs
   Vine-Ripened Tomato Salad
   1 baked sweet potato

Dessert
   Cinnamon Lemon Poached Pear with Cherry Syrup

Day 12

On Arising
Slim Chai Tea

Breakfast
2 hard-boiled eggs
1 tomato, sliced
Fresh grapefruit
Decaffeinated coffee with nonfat milk

Morning Snack
Blueberry Yogurt Cup
Slim Chai Tea

Lunch
Immune Power Soup
Herb Hummus Wrap
Slim Chai Tea

Afternoon Snack
Vegetable juice
12 raw almonds

Dinner
Walnut-Crusted Fish
Pomodori con Mozzarella (Tomatoes with Mozzarella)
2 cups mixed salad greens
1 tablespoon Pesto Vinaigrette

Dessert
Strawberry Mango Granita

Day 13

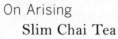

On Arising
   Slim Chai Tea

Breakfast
   Blueberry Cinnamon Bowl
   Fresh grapefruit
   Decaffeinated coffee with nonfat milk

Morning Snack
   Carrot and celery sticks with 1 teaspoon almond butter
   Slim Chai Tea

Lunch
   Asian Grilled Chicken Salad
   2 tablespoons Pomegranate Lime Dressing
   Slim Chai Tea

Afternoon Snack
   Vegetable juice
   12 raw almonds

Dinner
   Fifteen-Minute Chili
   served over ½ cup brown rice
   Garden Salad
   1 tablespoon Pesto Vinaigrette

Dessert
   Pineapple Orange Granita

Day 14

On Arising
   Slim Chai Tea

Breakfast
   Frittata with Tomato, Capers, and Cilantro
   Fresh orange
   Decaffeinated coffee with nonfat milk

Morning Snack
   1 cup broccoli florets
   Slim Chai Tea

Lunch
   Immune Power Soup
   Cottage Cheese with Apple and Walnuts
   Slim Chai Tea

Afternoon Snack
   Pomegranate juice
   12 raw almonds

Dinner
   Big Vegetable Bowl

Dessert
   Fried Bananas

Stage 2

~~~

Recipes

Breakfasts

OMEGA BLAST GRANOLA

STAGE 2

Granola is a crunchy and satisfying comfort food. This recipe has a great mix of whole-grain oats, fruit, and nuts, and is high in omega-3s. Make it in advance when you have a couple of minutes and then it's ready when you need it. This healthy granola is a delicious way to start your day.

    3 cups rolled oats
    1 cup oat bran
    ½ cup chopped walnuts
    ¼ cup freshly ground flaxseeds
    ¾ cup pomegranate juice
    2 teaspoons walnut oil or olive oil
    1 teaspoon cinnamon
    1 teaspoon vanilla
    1 cup raisins

Preheat the oven to 325°F. In a big bowl, mix everything except the raisins. Spread the mixture over a nonstick baking pan and bake for 20 minutes, or until nice and brown, stirring occasionally to cook evenly. Remove from the oven and toss in the raisins. Let cool and put in a glass container; store in the refrigerator. Makes about 5 cups. Serve 1 cup granola with 1 cup nonfat plain yogurt, nonfat milk, or unsweetened soymilk per person.

NUTRITION PER SERVING: 458 Calories | 13 g Protein | 78 g Carbohydrates | 15 g Fat

FRITTATA WITH TOMATO, CAPERS, AND CILANTRO

Olive oil spray

3 egg whites, lightly beaten

¼ teaspoon salt

Freshly ground black pepper

½ tomato, diced

2 tablespoons chopped fresh cilantro

1 tablespoon capers, rinsed

2 cups mixed salad greens

Heat a nonstick frying pan over medium heat and coat it with olive oil spray. Pour the egg whites into the pan and season with salt and pepper. Spread the tomato, cilantro, and capers evenly over the eggs and cook over medium heat for 4 minutes, or until the eggs are set. Turn the whole thing over and cook for 2 minutes more. Serve over a bed of mixed salad greens. Serves 1.

NUTRITION PER SERVING: 89 Calories | 12 g Protein | 7 g Carbohydrates | 2 g Fat

BLUEBERRY CINNAMON BOWL

An update on a morning tradition, here is a quick and easy hot breakfast. The aroma of blueberries and cinnamon rising from the bowl makes this a special treat. Oatmeal is a great source of cholesterol-lowering fiber, and cinnamon reduces insulin levels.

½ cup rolled oats
½ cup fresh or frozen blueberries
1 tablespoon freshly ground flaxseeds
½ tablespoon ground walnuts
Dash of cinnamon

Bring 1 cup water to a boil in a small saucepan, then stir in the oats. Cook for 4 minutes, then add the berries and cook until piping hot. Mix in the flaxseeds, walnuts, and cinnamon. Serves 1.

NUTRITION PER SERVING: 251 Calories | 9 g Protein | 40 g Carbohydrates | 7 g Fat

BANANA STRAWBERRY SMOOTHIE

1 cup nonfat plain yogurt
1 banana, sliced
½ cup fresh or frozen strawberries
1 tablespoon freshly ground flaxseeds
1 tablespoon whey protein concentrate

Pour 2 tablespoons water into a blender. Add the yogurt, banana, and strawberries and blend. Put in the ground flaxseeds and whey protein. Blend until smooth. Pour into a tall glass and enjoy! Serves 1.

NUTRITION PER SERVING: 332 Calories | 15 g Protein | 45 g Carbohydrates | 5 g Fat

Lunches

BASMATI RICE SALAD

STAGE 2

The big, bold flavors of fresh herbs and exotic spices make this a deeply satisfying dish.

1 cup cooked basmati rice

1 cup cooked or canned garbanzo beans (chickpeas),
   drained and rinsed

1 red, yellow, or green bell pepper, finely diced

½ cup chopped celery

2 tablespoons freshly ground flaxseeds

¼ cup finely chopped scallions

2 tablespoons chopped fresh parsley

2 teaspoons toasted sesame oil

Juice of 1 lemon

¼ teaspoon cumin

¼ teaspoon turmeric

¼ teaspoon salt

4 cups chopped arugula

1 teaspoon sesame seeds, for garnish

In a large bowl, combine the rice, garbanzos, pepper, celery, flaxseeds, scallions, and parsley. In a small bowl, whisk together the sesame oil and lemon juice, then add the cumin, turmeric, and salt. Pour the dressing over the salad and mix well. Serve over a bed of arugula and sprinkle with sesame seeds. Serves 2.

NUTRITION PER SERVING: 348 Calories | 11 g Protein | 57 g Carbohydrates | 10 g Fat

INSALATA CAPRESE
Mozzarella and Tomato Salad

Toss together a few simple ingredients to make this delightful salad. Basil has a fresh, robust flavor and is a powerful anti-inflammatory herb.

4 ounces sliced low-fat mozzarella cheese
1 tomato, diced
2 cups arugula or baby spinach
2 tablespoons chopped fresh basil
1 teaspoon extra virgin olive oil
1 teaspoon freshly ground flaxseeds
¼ teaspoon salt

Alternate sliced mozzarella with tomato on a bed of arugula. Top with the basil, extra virgin olive oil, flaxseeds, and salt. Serves 1.

NUTRITION PER SERVING: 292 Calories | 20 g Protein | 11 g Carbohydrates | 19 g Fat

TOFU "EGG" SALAD

This is a fun, easy way to enjoy tofu. Tofu egg salad gets its crunch from fresh vegetables and its bright color from turmeric, which has strong anti-inflammatory effects.

STAGE 2

One 14-ounce package firm or extra-firm tofu
½ carrot, finely diced
2 stalks scallions, finely chopped
2 tablespoons chopped fresh parsley
1 garlic clove, chopped
2 teaspoons capers, rinsed
Juice of ½ lemon
¼ teaspoon turmeric
2 cups mixed greens
¼ teaspoon salt
Freshly ground black pepper

Drain the tofu, rinse with cold water, and pat dry. Place the tofu in a large bowl and mash it with a fork. Toss in the carrot, scallions, parsley, garlic, and capers. Add the lemon juice and turmeric and mix well. Serve over mixed greens and season with salt and pepper. Serves 2.

NUTRITION PER SERVING: 132 Calories | 15 g Protein | 9 g Carbohydrates | 4 g Fat

SUMMER COOL CUCUMBER SOUP

STAGE 2

1 cucumber, peeled and seeded
2 cups nonfat plain yogurt
1 garlic clove, minced
1 teaspoon extra virgin olive oil
Juice of ½ lime
2 tablespoons chopped fresh mint

Chop the cucumber and put it in a blender with the yogurt, garlic, extra virgin olive oil, and lime juice. Blend until smooth. Add the chopped mint and mix again. Pour into bowls to serve. Serves 2.

NUTRITION PER SERVING: 88 Calories | 6 g Protein | 15 g Carbohydrates | 2 g Fat

WINTER WARM TOMATO BASIL SOUP

Because this soup is made without sugar, the wonderful tanginess of the tomato shines through. Fresh basil adds a hint of spiciness, while the turmeric gives it a mellow richness.

2 cups canned tomato puree
Shake of turmeric
Shake of garlic powder
Pinch of salt
Freshly ground black pepper
1 tablespoon chopped fresh basil

Put the tomato puree in a saucepan. Add 2 cups water, the turmeric, garlic powder, salt, and pepper. Bring to a boil, then lower the heat and simmer, uncovered, for 5 minutes, stirring often. Top with the basil and serve in bowls or mugs. Serves 2.

NUTRITION PER SERVING: 96 Calories | 4 g Protein | 22 g Carbohydrates | 0.5 g Fat

INSALATA FAGIOLI
Italian Bean Salad

One 15-ounce can cannellini beans
5 plum tomatoes, chopped
1 cucumber, peeled and chopped
½ red bell pepper, finely chopped
2 stalks scallions, finely chopped
1 tablespoon extra virgin olive oil
Juice of 1 lemon
¼ teaspoon turmeric
½ teaspoon salt
Freshly ground black pepper
½ cup finely chopped fresh parsley
4 cups arugula

Put the cannellini beans in a strainer and rinse with cold water. In a large bowl, mix the tomatoes, cucumber, bell pepper, and scallions. In a small bowl, whisk together the extra virgin olive oil, lemon juice, turmeric, salt, and pepper. Fold the beans into the vegetable mixture, add the dressing, and shower with fresh parsley. Serve over arugula. Serves 2.

NUTRITION PER SERVING: 306 Calories | 12 g Protein | 46 g Carbohydrates | 9 g Fat

CHICKEN CAESAR SALAD

STAGE 2

5 ounces cooked skinless, boneless chicken breast, cut into strips

3 cups chopped romaine lettuce

1 tomato, cut into wedges

2 anchovies, chopped

2 teaspoons grated Parmesan cheese or other hard cheese

Juice of ½ lemon

1 teaspoon walnut oil or extra virgin olive oil

Pinch of salt

Freshly ground black pepper

Mix the chicken, lettuce, tomato, and anchovies. Sprinkle with the Parmesan cheese. Whisk together the lemon juice, walnut oil, salt, and pepper and keep in a small container separate from the salad until ready to eat. Serves 1.

LUNCH TIP TO GO: Mix the salad directly in a take-away container, and you have a healthy lunch to go. Bring the salad dressing in a separate small container.

NUTRITION PER SERVING: 355 Calories | 58 g Protein | 8 g Carbohydrates | 10 g Fat

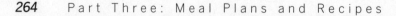

ASIAN GRILLED CHICKEN SALAD

Traditional Asian cuisine treasures the health-giving properties of fresh vegetables and spices. Scallions are prized in Chinese and Japanese cooking for their ability to boost the immune system. Sesame seeds are a good source of magnesium, a mineral needed for energy and muscle relaxation. Here the soy sauce imparts a hearty flavor to the chicken, while the fragrant scallions bring in a touch of spiciness.

2 tablespoons low-sodium soy sauce

1 tablespoon toasted sesame oil

Freshly ground black pepper

12 ounces skinless, boneless chicken breasts

Olive oil spray

1 cup torn lettuce or mixed salad greens

2 tablespoons chopped fresh cilantro

2 stalks scallions, chopped

½ teaspoon sesame seeds

Heat an electric grill or grill pan. In a bowl large enough to hold the chicken, mix the soy sauce, sesame oil, and pepper. Slice the chicken, coat it well with the mixture, and marinate, covered, in the refrigerator for 10 minutes. Spray the grill with olive oil. Remove the chicken from the marinade (dispose of the remaining marinade) and place it on the grill; cook over medium heat for 5 minutes total, turning often, or until cooked through. Remove the chicken and let cool. Spread the chicken over the lettuce, sprinkle with the cilantro, scallions, and sesame seeds, and enjoy. Serves 2.

NUTRITION PER SERVING: 230 Calories | 40 g Protein | 3 g Carbohydrates | 5 g Fat

HERB HUMMUS WRAP

2 tablespoons chopped fresh herbs: cilantro, chives, parsley, oregano,
  or basil
½ cup hummus
½ cup grated carrot
3 romaine lettuce leaves
¼ teaspoon salt
Freshly ground black pepper

Mix the herbs into the hummus. Spread some hummus and carrot on
each romaine leaf. Sprinkle with salt and pepper, then fold into a
wrap. Serves 1.

NUTRITION PER SERVING: 236 Calories | 11 g Protein | 24 g Carbohydrates | 16 g Fat

Dinners

APRICOT MINT CHICKEN

1 tablespoon whole wheat flour or all-purpose flour

¼ teaspoon salt

Freshly ground black pepper

Two 8-ounce skinless, boneless chicken breasts

Olive oil spray

1 onion, diced

4 garlic cloves, minced

4 cups baby spinach or one 10-ounce package frozen spinach,
    thawed and squeezed dry

10 dried apricot halves

12 fresh mint leaves, chopped

On a plate, mix the flour, salt, and pepper. Cut the chicken into cubes and dredge them in the flour mixture, coating the chicken.

Heat a nonstick skillet and coat it with olive oil spray. Put the chicken in the skillet and cook over medium heat for 5 minutes, turning to brown all sides. Add the onion and garlic and cook for 3 minutes. Add the spinach, apricots, and mint and cook for 4 minutes, stirring occasionally. Serves 2.

NUTRITION PER SERVING: 351 Calories | 55 g Protein | 23 g Carbohydrates | 4 g Fat

GINGER LIME GRILLED TUNA

Grilling perfectly accentuates the subtle flavors of tuna. In this recipe a quick ginger marinade gets the fish ready for the grill. Tuna is high in protein and rich in omega-3s. Ginger is used around the world for its flavor and contains dozens of inflammation-fighting phytonutrients called gingerols.

1 tablespoon peeled, minced fresh ginger or 1 teaspoon ground ginger
Juice of 1 lime
1 tablespoon low-sodium soy sauce
1 teaspoon extra virgin olive oil
Freshly ground black pepper
12 ounces tuna steak, 1 inch thick
Olive oil spray
¼ cup chopped fresh chives, for garnish

Whisk the ginger, lime juice, soy sauce, and extra virgin olive oil together in a shallow bowl. Add the pepper, then put the tuna in the bowl and turn to coat well. Cover the bowl and marinate the tuna in the refrigerator for 15 minutes.

Heat an electric grill or grill pan. Spray the grill with olive oil. Remove the tuna from the marinade and place on the grill. Dispose of the remaining marinade. Cook the tuna over medium-high heat for 2 minutes, then turn. Cook for another 2 minutes, or until the inside is a nice light pink. You want to take the tuna off the grill before it's well done, because it continues to cook even after it's off the heat. Garnish with chives. Serves 2.

NUTRITION PER SERVING: 267 Calories | 52 g Protein | 2 g Carbohydrates | 4 g Fat

GRILLED STEAK WITH CHIMICHURRI SAUCE

Chimichurri Sauce
½ red onion, finely diced
¼ cup finely chopped fresh cilantro
¼ cup finely chopped fresh parsley
1 teaspoon extra virgin olive oil
2 tablespoons vinegar
Juice of ½ lime

Grilled Steak
2 garlic cloves, minced
½ cup unsweetened pomegranate juice
12 ounces flank steak
¼ teaspoon salt
Freshly ground black pepper
Olive oil spray

To make the chimichurri sauce, combine the onion, cilantro, parsley, extra virgin olive oil, vinegar, and lime juice.

To make the marinade, mix the garlic and pomegranate juice in a shallow bowl. Add the flank steak and turn to coat both sides well, then season with salt and pepper. Heat an electric grill or grill pan and spray it with olive oil. Place the steak on the grill and cook over medium heat for 5 to 6 minutes on each side, until cooked through. Discard the marinade. Remove the steak from the heat and let rest for 5 minutes, then slice. To serve, top the steak with the chimichurri sauce. Serves 2.

NUTRITION PER SERVING: 433 Calories | 48 g Protein | 10 g Carbohydrates | 21 g Fat

GINGER INFUSED SALMON

STAGE 2

Two 8-ounce salmon fillets

Olive oil spray

½ cup peeled, julienned fresh ginger

1 bunch scallions, cut lengthwise into matchstick-sized pieces

1 tablespoon low-sodium soy sauce

Rinse the salmon with cold water and pat dry with a paper towel. Heat a nonstick skillet with a lid and coat with olive oil spray. Place the salmon in the skillet and cook for 1 to 2 minutes over medium-high heat, then turn the fish over. Top with the ginger and scallions. Pour the soy sauce into the bottom of the pan, cover, and steam for 6 minutes, or until the center of the salmon turns from red to pink. Plate the salmon with the ginger and scallions on top. Serves 2.

NUTRITION PER SERVING: 367 Calories | 46 g Protein | 10 g Carbohydrates | 15 g Fat

ROASTED SALMON WITH GINGER, GARLIC, AND SCALLIONS

This is a great way to cook salmon right in your toaster oven. The top gets golden brown and the scallions get nice and crunchy. Ginger, garlic, and scallions enhance the flavor of the salmon and also contain protective phytonutrients.

Olive oil spray

Two 8-ounce salmon fillets

2 stalks scallions

1 garlic clove, crushed

2 tablespoons peeled, minced fresh ginger

¼ teaspoon salt

Freshly ground black pepper

Juice of ½ lime

Preheat the toaster oven to 375°F and spray a baking pan with olive oil. Rinse the salmon with cold water and pat dry with a paper towel. Cut the scallions into 4-inch sticks and then slice lengthwise. Place the salmon on the baking pan and spread the scallions, garlic, and ginger across the top. Season with salt and pepper, then bake for 4 minutes. Switch the oven to broil and cook for 3 to 4 minutes more, until the center of the salmon turns from red to pink. Finish with a sprinkle of lime juice. Serves 2.

NUTRITION PER SERVING: 339 Calories | 45 g Protein | 4 g Carbohydrates | 14 g Fat

STIR-FRIED VEGETABLES
WITH BEEF OR TOFU

STAGE 2

6 ounces stir-fry beef or flank steak or one 14-ounce package
firm or extra-firm tofu

Freshly ground black pepper

Olive oil spray

1 teaspoon toasted sesame oil

3 garlic cloves, minced

½ onion, diced

2 carrots, sliced into rounds

3 cups broccoli florets

1 cup sliced shiitake or white button mushrooms

2 tablespoons low-sodium soy sauce

1 teaspoon sesame seeds, for garnish

FOR BEEF

Cut the beef into ½-inch strips and season with pepper. Heat a non-stick frying pan or wok and coat with olive oil spray. Place the strips of beef in the pan and cook over medium heat for 2 to 3 minutes, until the meat is done. Transfer the meat to a bowl.

FOR TOFU

Cut the tofu into ¼-inch-thick slices and season with pepper. Heat a nonstick frying pan or wok and coat with olive oil spray. Put the tofu in the pan and cook over medium heat for 2 to 3 minutes on each side, until light brown and crispy. Transfer the tofu to a bowl.

To prepare the vegetables, heat a nonstick frying pan or wok and coat with the sesame oil. Put the garlic, onion, and carrots in the pan and cook over medium heat for 3 minutes. Add the broccoli and mush-rooms and cook for 5 minutes, stirring frequently. Return the cooked beef or tofu to the pan and mix with the vegetables, then remove from the heat. Sprinkle with soy sauce and sesame seeds and serve in bowls. Serves 2.

BEEF: NUTRITION PER SERVING: 358 Calories | 33 g Protein | 37 g Carbohydrates | 10 g Fat   **TOFU:** NUTRITION PER SERVING: 423 Calories | 37 g Protein | 45 g Car-bohydrates | 13 g Fat

STAGE

TERIYAKI CHICKEN

STAGE 2

⅓ cup low-sodium soy sauce

Juice of 1 orange

2 garlic cloves, minced

1 tablespoon peeled, minced fresh ginger

Two 8-ounce skinless, boneless chicken breasts

Olive oil spray

¼ cup chopped fresh cilantro, for garnish

In a small saucepan, combine the soy sauce and orange juice. Bring to a boil, reduce the heat, and simmer over medium heat until the sauce thickens, about 10 minutes. Pour the mixture into a shallow bowl and mix in the garlic and ginger. Place the chicken in the bowl and coat well with the marinade. Cover the bowl and marinate in the refrigerator for 20 minutes. Meanwhile, preheat the oven to 400°F.

Spray a baking pan lightly with olive oil and place the chicken in the pan. Spoon some garlic and ginger pieces from the marinade over the chicken, and discard the remaining marinade. Put the chicken in the oven and roast for 15 minutes. This browns the chicken nicely. Then turn the oven down to 350°F and roast for 15 minutes more, or until the chicken is cooked through. Garnish with fresh cilantro. Serves 2.

NUTRITION PER SERVING: 183 Calories | 33 g Protein | 6 g Carbohydrates | 2 g Fat

FIFTEEN-MINUTE CHILI

One night I needed a healthy meal in a hurry, so I created this Fifteen-Minute Chili. Canned beans and tomato puree are quick and easy, and they taste great. With protein and fiber from the beans, lycopene from the tomatoes, and inflammation-fighting turmeric and cumin, this dish is loaded with key nutrients. You will love the cooking time and your friends and family will love the taste.

STAGE 2

One 15-ounce can kidney beans
One 15-ounce can black beans
1 tablespoon extra virgin olive oil
1 onion, diced
3 garlic cloves, minced
1 teaspoon cumin
¼ teaspoon turmeric
½ teaspoon salt
Freshly ground black pepper
One 15-ounce can tomato puree
½ cup chopped fresh parsley or cilantro, for garnish

Put the beans in a strainer and give them a quick rinse with cold water. Put the extra virgin olive oil in a large pot, then add the onion and garlic. Cook for 3 minutes over medium heat, then add the beans. Add the cumin, turmeric, salt, and pepper and cook for 2 minutes, letting the flavor get into the beans. Add the tomato puree and let the chili come to a boil, stirring often. Simmer for 5 minutes, then serve in bowls with a generous sprinkle of fresh parsley. Serves 4.

NUTRITION PER SERVING: 291 Calories | 14 g Protein | 53 g Carbohydrates | 4 g Fat

Sides and Dressings

GINGER ORANGE DRESSING

Juice of 1 orange

1 teaspoon walnut oil or extra virgin olive oil

1 teaspoon peeled, minced fresh ginger

Pinch of salt

Freshly ground black pepper

In a small bowl, whisk together the orange juice and walnut oil. Mix in the fresh ginger, salt, and pepper. Serves 2.

NUTRITION PER SERVING: 83 Calories | 0.6 g Protein | 9 g Carbohydrates | 5 g Fat

EGGPLANT TART

2 tablespoons low-fat goat cheese

4 slices eggplant, ¼ inch thick

8 walnut halves

4 cherry tomatoes, halved

2 tablespoons chopped fresh herbs of your choice

Pinch of salt

Olive oil spray

Preheat the toaster oven to 375°F. Spread some of the goat cheese on each eggplant slice. Add 2 walnut halves and 2 cherry tomato halves to each. Sprinkle with herbs and salt. Spray a baking pan with olive oil and place the eggplant slices in the pan. Bake until the eggplant softens and the cheese is golden brown, about 12 minutes. Serves 2.

NUTRITION PER SERVING: 110 Calories | 4 g Protein | 6 g Carbohydrates | 8 g Fat

ZUCCHINI WITH GARLIC AND HERBS

STAGE 2

1 teaspoon extra virgin olive oil

2 garlic cloves, minced

3 zucchini, diced

Pinch of salt

2 tablespoons finely chopped fresh parsley, for garnish

4 basil leaves, chopped, for garnish

Heat a nonstick skillet. Add the extra virgin olive oil and garlic and cook for 2 minutes over medium heat. Add the zucchini and salt and sauté for 5 minutes, stirring occasionally. Remove from the heat and sprinkle the parsley and basil on top. Serves 2.

NUTRITION PER SERVING: 55 Calories | 2 g Protein | 11 g Carbohydrates | 1 g Fat

LEMON SPICE DRESSING

Juice of 1 lemon

⅛ teaspoon cumin

⅛ teaspoon turmeric

⅛ teaspoon garlic powder

Pinch of salt

Freshly ground black pepper

2 teaspoons walnut oil or extra virgin olive oil

In a small bowl, whisk together the lemon juice, cumin, turmeric, and garlic powder. Add the salt, pepper, and walnut oil and whisk until well blended. Serves 2.

NUTRITION PER SERVING: 50 Calories | 0.15 g Protein | 2.5 g Carbohydrates | 4.5 g Fat

VINE-RIPENED TOMATO SALAD

1 vine-ripened tomato, diced

½ cucumber, diced

½ red, yellow, or green bell pepper, finely diced

¼ cup finely diced red onion

2 tablespoons chopped fresh parsley

Juice of ½ lime

1 teaspoon walnut oil or extra virgin olive oil

Pinch of salt

Freshly ground black pepper

Toss together the tomato, cucumber, bell pepper, onion, and parsley. Pour the lime juice and walnut oil over the top, season with salt and pepper, and mix to coat the salad with dressing. Serves 1.

NUTRITION PER SERVING: 121 Calories | 3 g Protein | 18 g Carbohydrates | 5 g Fat

Desserts

PINEAPPLE ORANGE GRANITA

STAGE 2

You can whip up this beautiful frosty dessert in minutes. The pineapple and orange taste like sunshine.

1 cup chopped pineapple, fresh or canned
¼ cup orange juice
1½ cups ice cubes

Puree the pineapple and orange juice in a blender. Add the ice and blend until smooth. Serve immediately or store in the freezer. For later use, remove from the freezer and let thaw until soft enough to break up with a fork. Serves 1.

NUTRITION PER SERVING: 102 Calories | 1 g Protein | 26 g Carbohydrates | 0.31 g Fat

WARM SPICED APRICOTS AND FIGS

1 teaspoon cinnamon
½ teaspoon cardamom
8 dried apricots, chopped
8 dried figs, chopped
Juice of ½ lemon

In a small saucepan, bring 1 cup water to a boil, then stir in the cinnamon and cardamom. Add the apricots and figs and simmer over low heat for 15 minutes. Remove with a slotted spoon to dessert bowls, ladle the juice on top, then sprinkle with lemon juice. Serves 4.

NUTRITION PER SERVING: 135 Calories | 2 g Protein | 34 g Carbohydrates | 0.3 g Fat

FRIED BANANAS

Cooking really brings out an incredible sweetness in the bananas, so you can enjoy this tropical dessert without added sugar.

Olive oil spray
2 yellow bananas, sliced lengthwise
Juice of ½ lemon
Sprinkle of cinnamon

Heat a nonstick frying pan over medium heat and coat with olive oil spray. Place the banana slices cut side down in the pan. Cook for 3 to 4 minutes on each side, until the bananas are slightly caramelized. Plate the bananas and finish with the lemon juice and a sprinkle of cinnamon. Serves 2.

NUTRITION PER SERVING: 113 Calories | 1.33 g Protein | 27 g Carbohydrates | 0.97 g Fat

Stage 3

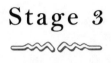

Meal Plan

Stage 3 is the ultimate maintenance program. The Fat Resistance Foods that helped you lose weight in Stage 1 and Stage 2 are back to keep inflammation down, allowing you to maintain your target weight. What's more, these foods can make you look and feel younger, help prevent cancer, boost your immune system, and keep you healthy. With whole-grain breads and pastas, this stage offers meals that are fun and easy to prepare. Recipes such as Blueberry Flax Pancakes, Carrot Raisin Muffins, and Shrimp Scampi with Linguine make following the Stage 3 meal plan a pleasure. Emphasizing variety and choice, we have included vegetarian meals such as Minestrone Rustica and Vegetarian Curry. We wish you a lifetime of good health and good eating.

Day 1

On Arising
  Slim Chai Tea

Breakfast
  Blueberry Flax Pancakes
  Fresh grapefruit
  Decaffeinated coffee with nonfat milk

Morning Snack
  1 cup broccoli florets
  Slim Chai Tea

Lunch
  Hummus and Greens on Tortilla
  Slim Chai Tea

Afternoon Snack
  Vegetable juice

Dinner
  Crabcakes with Tropical Salsa
  2 cups steamed green beans with lemon juice and
    ¼ cup slivered raw almonds

Dessert
  Pomegranate Banana Parfait

Day 2

On Arising
  Slim Chai Tea

Breakfast
  Smoked Salmon Frittata
  Fresh grapefruit
  Decaffeinated coffee with nonfat milk

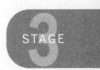

Morning Snack
  8 walnut halves
  Slim Chai Tea

Lunch
  Penne with Cherry Tomatoes and Ricotta
  2 cups arugula
  1 tablespoon Pesto Vinaigrette
  Slim Chai Tea

Afternoon Snack
  Iced Mocha Latte

Dinner
  Spinach Leek Soup
  Grilled Sirloin with Garlic and Herbs
  Vine-Ripened Tomato Salad

Dessert
  Cinnamon Lemon Poached Pear with Cherry Syrup

Day 3

STAGE 3

On Arising
  Slim Chai Tea

Breakfast
  Carrot Raisin Muffins
  Fresh grapefruit
  Decaffeinated coffee with nonfat milk

Morning Snack
  1 red or yellow bell pepper, sliced
  Slim Chai Tea

Lunch
  Immune Power Soup
  Chicken Caesar Salad
  Slim Chai Tea

Afternoon Snack
  Vegetable juice
  12 raw almonds

Dinner
  Pasta with Tuscan White Beans
  Zucchini with Garlic and Herbs

Dessert
  Strawberry Mango Granita

Day 4

On Arising
    Slim Chai Tea

Breakfast
    Your Favorite Omelet
    Fresh orange
    Decaffeinated coffee with nonfat milk

Morning Snack
    8 walnut halves
    Slim Chai Tea

Lunch
    Melted Cheese and Fresh Herb Panini
    Slim Chai Tea

Afternoon Snack
    Vegetable juice
    12 raw almonds

Dinner
    Sesame-Crusted Grilled Tuna with Caramelized Onion
    Asparagus with Red Bell Pepper and Garlic
    Oven-Roasted Rosemary Potatoes

Dessert
    Baked Apple with Cinnamon and Walnuts

Day 5

STAGE 3

On Arising
   Slim Chai Tea

Breakfast
   Omega Blast Granola with 1 cup nonfat plain yogurt,
      nonfat milk, or unsweetened soymilk and ½ apple,
      chopped
   Decaffeinated coffee with nonfat milk

Morning Snack
   Carrot and celery sticks
   Slim Chai Tea

Lunch
   Turkey and Cheese Sandwich
   Slim Chai Tea

Afternoon Snack
   Pomegranate juice
   12 almonds

Dinner
   Immune Power Soup
   Grilled Vegetables with Tofu
      served over ½ cup brown rice

Dessert
   Pineapple Orange Granita

Day 6

On Arising
  Slim Chai Tea

Breakfast
  Breakfast Burrito
  Fresh orange
  Decaffeinated coffee with nonfat milk

Morning Snack
  1 cup broccoli florets
  Slim Chai Tea

Lunch
  Baby Spinach Salad with Apple and Roasted Walnuts
  2 tablespoons Pomegranate Lime Dressing
  Slim Chai Tea

Afternoon Snack
  Vegetable juice
  12 raw almonds

Dinner
  Chicken and Peppers
  ½ cup brown rice
  Garden Salad
  1 teaspoon each extra virgin olive oil and lemon juice

Dessert
  Blueberry Parfait

Day 7

STAGE
3

On Arising
   Slim Chai Tea

Breakfast
   Smart Start Smoothie
   Fresh orange
   Decaffeinated coffee with nonfat milk

Morning Snack
   1 cup broccoli florets
   Slim Chai Tea

Lunch
   Orzo Salad
   Slim Chai Tea

Afternoon Snack
   Vegetable juice
   12 raw almonds

Dinner
   Spinach Leek Soup
   Roasted Salmon with Ginger, Garlic, and Scallions
   Eggplant Tart

Dessert
   Cherry Mint Parfait

Day 8

On Arising
   Slim Chai Tea

Breakfast
   Grandma's Apple Pancakes with Blueberry Syrup
   Decaffeinated coffee with nonfat milk

Morning Snack
   Carrot and celery sticks
   Slim Chai Tea

Lunch
   Salmon Salad
   Slim Chai Tea

Afternoon Snack
   Pomegranate juice

Dinner
   Apricot Mint Chicken
   Oven-Roasted Rosemary Potatoes
   2 cups mixed salad greens
   1 teaspoon each extra virgin olive oil and lemon juice

Dessert
   Frosty Yogurt with 12 crushed raw almonds

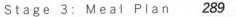

Day 9

On Arising
  Slim Chai Tea

Breakfast
  Frittata with Tomato, Capers, and Cilantro
  Fresh orange
  Decaffeinated coffee with nonfat milk

STAGE 3

Morning Snack
  8 walnut halves
  Slim Chai Tea

Lunch
  Portobello Pizza con Ricotta
  2 cups mixed salad greens
  1 tablespoon Lemon Spice Dressing
  Slim Chai Tea

Afternoon Snack
  Blueberry Yogurt Cup
    with 12 crushed raw almonds

Dinner
  Spinach Leek Soup
  Herb-Crusted Fish
  Corn and Tomato Salsa

Dessert
  Black Forest Banana Split

Day 10

On Arising
  Slim Chai Tea

Breakfast
  Papaya with Yogurt and Berries
  Decaffeinated coffee with nonfat milk

Morning Snack
  Carrot and celery sticks with 1 teaspoon almond butter
  Slim Chai Tea

Lunch
  Smoked Salmon on Whole-Grain Bread
  Slim Chai Tea

Afternoon Snack
  Vegetable juice
  12 raw almonds

Dinner
  Chicken Quesadilla with Tomato Salsa
  2 cups mixed salad greens
  1 teaspoon each extra virgin olive oil and lemon juice

Dessert
  Strawberry Mango Granita

Day 11

On Arising
    Slim Chai Tea

Breakfast
    Pizza Frittata
    Fresh orange
    Decaffeinated coffee with nonfat milk

Morning Snack
    1 cup broccoli florets
    Slim Chai Tea

Lunch
    Tofu "Egg" Salad
    Whole wheat pita
    Slim Chai Tea

Afternoon Snack
    Pomegranate juice
    12 raw almonds

Dinner
    Seared Scallops
    2 cups mixed salad greens
    1 teaspoon each extra virgin olive oil and lemon juice
    1 baked sweet potato

Dessert
    Kiwi Crunch Parfait

STAGE 3

Day 12

On Arising
   Slim Chai Tea

Breakfast
   Carrot Raisin Muffins
   Decaffeinated coffee with nonfat milk

STAGE

Morning Snack
   Blueberry Yogurt Cup
   Slim Chai Tea

Lunch
   Spicy Tuna on Whole-Grain Bread
   Slim Chai Tea

Afternoon Snack
   Vegetable juice
   12 raw almonds

Dinner
   Minestrone Rustica
   Garden Salad
   1 tablespoon Pesto Vinaigrette

Dessert
   Fried Bananas

Day 13

STAGE 3

On Arising
  Slim Chai Tea

Breakfast
  Breakfast Burrito
  Fresh orange
  Decaffeinated coffee with nonfat milk

Morning Snack
  1 red or yellow bell pepper, sliced
  Slim Chai Tea

Lunch
  Immune Power Soup
  Baby Spinach Salad with Apple and Roasted Walnuts
  1 tablespoon Pomegranate Lime Dressing
  Slim Chai Tea

Afternoon Snack
  Vegetable juice
  12 raw almonds

Dinner
  Shrimp Scampi with Linguine
  2 cups arugula
  1 teaspoon each extra virgin olive oil and lemon juice

Dessert
  1 cup fresh strawberries

Day 14

On Arising
    Slim Chai Tea

Breakfast
    Banana Strawberry Smoothie
    Decaffeinated coffee with nonfat milk

Morning Snack
    Carrot and celery sticks with 1 teaspoon almond butter
    Slim Chai Tea

Lunch
    Melted Cheese and Fresh Herb Panini
    Slim Chai Tea

Afternoon Snack
    Iced Mocha Latte
    12 raw almonds

Dinner
    Immune Power Soup
    Chicken Curry or Vegetarian Curry,
        served over ½ cup brown rice

Dessert
    Pineapple Orange Granita

Stage 3

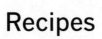

Recipes

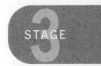

Breakfasts

BLUEBERRY FLAX PANCAKES

Bursting with blueberries, these pancakes make a nice family breakfast or weekend brunch.

STAGE 3

2 egg whites

¾ cup nonfat milk or unsweetened soymilk

1 tablespoon walnut oil

¾ cup whole wheat flour

¼ cup soy flour

1 tablespoon freshly ground flaxseeds

½ teaspoon baking powder

1 cup fresh or frozen blueberries, thawed

Olive oil spray

In a large bowl, whisk together the egg whites, milk, and walnut oil. Combine the whole wheat flour, soy flour, flaxseeds, and baking powder in another bowl. Add the dry ingredients to the wet ingredients and stir just until combined. Gently fold the blueberries into the batter.

Heat a griddle or frying pan and coat lightly with olive oil spray. When a drop of water bounces off the surface, the pan is ready. Using a tablespoon, drop the batter onto the griddle. Cook over medium heat for 3 minutes, then flip the pancakes over and press down to flatten. Cook on the other side for 4 minutes, or until golden brown and cooked through. The batter should make 8 pancakes. Serves 2.

NUTRITION PER SERVING: 376 Calories | 18 g Protein | 54 g Carbohydrates | 12 g Fat

CARROT RAISIN MUFFINS

It's exciting to make a tasty muffin using only healthy ingredients. These muffins have just a touch of sweetness and a satisfying chewiness. Perfect for breakfast on the go, they contain protein, fiber, omega-3s, and inflammation-fighting carotenoids.

1¼ cups whole wheat flour

½ cup soy flour

½ cup oat bran

⅓ cup chopped walnuts

¾ cup raisins

1½ teaspoons baking powder

1 teaspoon cinnamon

¼ cup freshly ground flaxseeds

¼ teaspoon salt

3 egg whites, lightly beaten

½ cup canned crushed pineapple, drained

½ cup walnut oil

2 cups grated carrots

In a large bowl, mix the whole wheat flour, soy flour, oat bran, walnuts, raisins, baking powder, cinnamon, flaxseeds, and salt. In another bowl, combine the egg whites, pineapple, walnut oil, and carrots. Fold the wet ingredients into the dry ingredients. Add 2 tablespoons water, or enough to make the batter workable: it's going to be thick. Line a muffin tin with cupcake liners and spoon the batter into the liners. The batter should almost fill each liner. Bake for 35 minutes, or until the muffins are cooked through. Makes 12. One serving is 2 muffins.

NUTRITION PER SERVING: 394 Calories | 14 g Protein | 50 g Carbohydrates | 19 g Fat

BREAKFAST BURRITO

This breakfast burrito is a tasty and fun way to get lots of nutrition for breakfast. Cilantro and scallions contain antioxidants and are anti-inflammatory. Egg whites supply high-quality protein. Yogurt and cheese supply calcium, which promotes weight loss.

STAGE 3

Olive oil spray
2 tablespoons chopped scallions
1 garlic clove, minced
3 egg whites, lightly beaten
¼ teaspoon salt
Freshly ground black pepper
1 whole wheat tortilla
1 ounce low-fat Cheddar cheese, chopped
1 tomato, chopped
2 tablespoons chopped fresh cilantro or parsley
2 tablespoons nonfat plain yogurt

Heat a small nonstick frying pan. Coat the pan with olive oil spray, add the scallions and garlic, and cook for 1 to 2 minutes over medium heat. Pour the egg whites over the scallions and garlic. Season with salt and pepper. Cook for 4 minutes, or until the eggs are set. Flip the eggs and cook for 2 minutes more. Remove from the heat, cut the eggs into strips, and spread across the tortilla. Add the cheese, tomato, and cilantro, then roll the tortilla to form a burrito. Add a dollop of yogurt on the side. Serves 1.

NUTRITION PER SERVING: 239 Calories | 24 g Protein | 32 g Carbohydrates | 4 g Fat

GRANDMA'S APPLE PANCAKES
WITH BLUEBERRY SYRUP

These pancakes are an original family recipe. The batter turns a beautiful golden brown as it cooks, while the apple inside gets soft and warm. The whole grain and apple make these pancakes a satisfying and nutritious meal. Absolutely simple and easy to make, this recipe lets you indulge in pancakes the healthy way.

3 egg whites

¼ cup nonfat milk or unsweetened soymilk

½ cup whole wheat flour

½ cup soy flour

½ cup crushed walnuts

2 apples

Olive oil spray

2 teaspoons blueberry concentrate

In a large bowl, lightly beat the egg whites. Add the milk, then stir in the whole wheat flour, soy flour, and walnuts. Peel and core the apples and slice them into rounds. The idea is to get them nice and thin.

Heat a griddle or frying pan and lightly coat it with olive oil spray. One by one, dip the apple rounds in the batter until completely covered, then place them on the hot pan. Cook, turning once, until golden brown on both sides. Serve with blueberry concentrate as syrup. Serves 2.

NUTRITION PER SERVING: 457 Calories | 20 g Protein | 59 g Carbohydrates | 15 g Fat

PAPAYA WITH YOGURT AND BERRIES

Enjoy the refreshing taste of the tropics with this quick and easy breakfast. Papaya is a good source of anti-inflammatory carotenoids, while yogurt provides protein and calcium.

½ papaya, seeded
Juice of ½ lime
1 cup nonfat plain yogurt
½ cup fresh blueberries or raspberries
8 walnut halves

Shower the halved papaya with lime juice and fill it with yogurt. Spoon the berries and walnuts over the top and enjoy. Serves 1.

NUTRITION PER SERVING: 282 Calories | 13 g Protein | 46 g Carbohydrates | 7 g Fat

PIZZA FRITTATA

Olive oil spray
1 garlic clove, minced
3 egg whites, lightly beaten
¼ cup shredded low-fat mozzarella cheese
½ tomato, sliced
2 tablespoons chopped fresh basil
¼ teaspoon salt
Freshly ground black pepper
2 cups arugula

Heat a small nonstick frying pan. Coat the pan with olive oil spray, add the garlic, and cook for 1 to 2 minutes over medium heat. Pour the egg whites over the garlic, then spread the mozzarella, tomato, and basil over the eggs. Season with salt and pepper. Cook for 4 minutes, or until the eggs are set. Flip the frittata over and cook for 2 minutes more. Remove from the pan and cut into quarters, like pizza slices. Place over a bed of arugula. Serves 1.

NUTRITION PER SERVING: 172 Calories | 19 g Protein | 8 g Carbohydrates | 7 g Fat

Lunches

HUMMUS AND GREENS ON TORTILLA

¼ cup hummus

1 whole wheat tortilla

2 cups mixed salad greens

4 cherry tomatoes, halved

1 garlic clove, minced

2 stalks scallions, chopped

Pinch of salt

Freshly ground black pepper

Spread the hummus evenly across the tortilla, then add the mixed salad greens, tomatoes, garlic, and scallions. Season with salt and pepper. Roll up to form a wrap. Serves 1.

NUTRITION PER SERVING: 224 Calories | 10 g Protein | 38 g Carbohydrates | 7 g Fat

TURKEY AND CHEESE SANDWICH

4 ounces sliced turkey breast

1 slice low-fat cheese

2 slices whole wheat or whole-grain bread

½ tomato, sliced

1 lettuce leaf

Makes one sandwich. If you tuck the tomato between the turkey and cheese, the bread won't get soggy. Serves 1.

NUTRITION PER SERVING: 389 Calories | 48 g Protein | 32 g Carbohydrates | 8 g Fat

PENNE WITH CHERRY TOMATOES AND RICOTTA

½ cup cooked whole wheat penne (or any whole wheat pasta)

1 cup cherry or grape tomatoes, halved

½ cup low-fat ricotta cheese

2 tablespoons chopped fresh basil

1 garlic clove, minced

¼ teaspoon salt

Freshly ground black pepper

2 cups arugula or mixed salad greens

1 teaspoon extra virgin olive oil

STAGE 3

Combine the penne, tomatoes, ricotta, basil, garlic, salt, and pepper. Serve over a bed of arugula, in a bowl or take-away container. Drizzle with extra virgin olive oil. Serves 1.

NUTRITION PER SERVING: 548 Calories | 23 g Protein | 99 g Carbohydrates | 7 g Fat

SALMON SALAD

3 cups mixed salad greens

6 cherry or grape tomatoes, halved

2 stalks scallions, chopped

2 tablespoons chopped fresh basil

½ grapefruit, peeled and diced

1 teaspoon extra virgin olive oil

Pinch of salt

Freshly ground black pepper

6 ounces cooked salmon

Toss the mixed salad greens, tomatoes, scallions, basil, and grapefruit. Dress with extra virgin olive oil, salt, and pepper. Plate the salmon on top of the salad. Serves 1.

NUTRITION PER SERVING: 382 Calories | 38 g Protein | 21 g Carbohydrates | 16 g Fat

MELTED CHEESE AND FRESH HERB PANINI

This is a really nice combination of inflammation-fighting fresh herbs and old-fashioned melted cheese.

STAGE 3

2 thin slices multigrain or whole wheat bread

3 ounces sliced low-fat cheese: Cheddar, mozzarella, or Swiss

1 garlic clove, minced

2 slices onion

½ tomato, sliced

½ cup chopped watercress

2 tablespoons chopped fresh herbs: basil, parsley, cilantro, sage, or dill

¼ teaspoon salt

Cover each slice of bread with cheese, garlic, and onion, then toast in a toaster oven until the cheese melts and turns golden brown. Add the tomato, watercress, herbs, and salt to one slice and place the other slice on top. Serves 1.

NUTRITION PER SERVING: 286 Calories | 28 g Protein | 31 g Carbohydrates | 8 g Fat

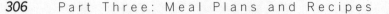

ORZO SALAD

Orzo is a delightful pasta that combines beautifully with fresh vegetables and herbs. This rice-shaped pasta can be found in the dry pasta section of the supermarket, and comes in a small box or bag.

STAGE

½ cup cooked orzo (or other pasta shape)
1 tomato, diced
½ cup diced low-fat mozzarella cheese
2 cups chopped arugula
½ cup sliced mushrooms
2 stalks scallions, chopped
1 garlic clove, minced
¼ teaspoon salt
Freshly ground black pepper
1 teaspoon extra virgin olive oil
2 tablespoons chopped fresh basil, for garnish

In a bowl or take-away container, toss the orzo, tomato, mozzarella, arugula, mushrooms, scallions, garlic, salt, and pepper. Finish with a drizzle of extra virgin olive oil and a sprinkle of basil. Serves 1.

NUTRITION PER SERVING: 485 Calories | 29 g Protein | 59 g Carbohydrates | 19 g Fat

SMOKED SALMON ON WHOLE-GRAIN BREAD

Smoked salmon makes eating healthy a pleasure. Nothing could be easier than this sandwich, which combines the rich flavor of salmon with the heartiness of whole-grain bread. Capers add a touch of tangy freshness.

STAGE

4 ounces sliced smoked salmon

½ tomato, sliced

2 slices onion

1 tablespoon capers, rinsed

2 slices whole-grain bread

Spread the salmon, tomato, onion, and capers over one slice of bread, then cover with the other slice. Cut the sandwich in half and enjoy. Serves 1.

NUTRITION PER SERVING: 277 Calories | 28 g Protein | 28 g Carbohydrates | 7 g Fat

SPICY TUNA ON WHOLE-GRAIN BREAD

This sandwich gets its fresh flavors from basil and lemon and its spice from scallions. Tuna is rich in omega-3s, and the vegetables have inflammation-fighting phytonutrients. Whole-grain bread means good complex carbohydrates.

One 6-ounce can water-packed tuna, drained
2 stalks scallions, chopped
2 tablespoons chopped fresh basil
Juice of ½ lemon or lime
1 teaspoon extra virgin olive oil
Shake of turmeric
Pinch of salt
Freshly ground black pepper
2 slices whole-grain bread
2 slices tomato

Mix the tuna, scallions, basil, lemon juice, extra virgin olive oil, turmeric, salt, and pepper. Spread the tuna mixture over one slice of bread, then top with the tomato and the second slice of bread.

NUTRITION PER SERVING: 397 Calories | 50 g Protein | 31 g Carbohydrates | 8 g Fat

STAGE 3

Dinners

CRABCAKES WITH TROPICAL SALSA

This recipe shows you how to enjoy a traditional favorite using healthy ingredients. These crabcakes, along with a tropical salsa that adds an exotic touch, can be put together quickly. Mango is a rich source of antioxidant flavonoids, which give it a distinctive orange color.

Crabcakes

2 potatoes, diced

2 egg whites, lightly beaten

2 stalks scallions, chopped

¼ cup chopped fresh parsley

¼ teaspoon salt

Freshly ground black pepper

6 ounces fresh or frozen lump crabmeat

Olive oil spray

Tropical Salsa

1 ripe mango, chopped

½ cup chopped fresh or canned pineapple

½ cup chopped red bell pepper

¼ cup finely chopped red onion

Juice of 1 lime

¼ cup finely chopped fresh cilantro

Bring a pot of water to a boil and add the potatoes. Boil for 8 minutes, or until fork-tender. Transfer the potatoes to a large bowl and mash. Mix in the egg whites, scallions, parsley, salt, and pepper. Check the crabmeat for shells and fold it into the potato mixture. Heat a nonstick frying pan over medium heat and coat it with olive oil spray.

Form the crabmeat mixture into small round patties and place them in the pan. Cook for 4 minutes each side, or until golden brown and cooked through.

For the salsa, combine the mango, pineapple, pepper, and onion in a bowl. Add the lime juice and cilantro and mix well. Plate the salsa next to the crabcakes. Serves 2.

STAGE

NUTRITION PER SERVING: 315 Calories | 22 g Protein | 53 g Carbohydrates | 2 g Fat

PASTA WITH TUSCAN WHITE BEANS

Enjoy the authentic Italian flavors in pasta, tomatoes, and garlic with this healthy recipe. Whole wheat pasta has protein and fiber, and tomatoes have lycopene.

1 teaspoon extra virgin olive oil

2 garlic cloves, chopped

1 cup canned cannellini beans

One 15-ounce can crushed tomatoes

½ teaspoon salt

Freshly ground black pepper

¼ cup chopped fresh basil

½ pound whole wheat penne or ziti (or any whole wheat pasta)

Heat a saucepan over medium heat, add the extra virgin olive oil and garlic, and sauté for 2 minutes. Rinse the beans with cold water, drain, and add them to the saucepan. Cook over medium heat for 4 minutes. Add the tomatoes, salt, and pepper and cook for 5 minutes. Remove from the heat and mix the basil into the tomatoes and beans.

While the beans are cooking, cook the penne. Fill a large pot halfway with cold water and bring it to a boil. When the water boils, add the pasta and cook for 7 to 10 minutes over high heat or according to directions on package. Test the pasta and remove when al dente, or soft enough to eat but still firm. Drain the pasta and mix with the tomato–bean sauce. Serves 2.

NUTRITION PER SERVING: 589 Calories | 25 g Protein | 120 g Carbohydrates | 5 g Fat

SESAME-CRUSTED GRILLED TUNA
WITH CARAMELIZED ONION

Grilled Tuna
Juice of 2 limes
1 tablespoon toasted sesame oil
Pinch of salt
Freshly ground black pepper
12 ounces tuna steak
¼ cup sesame seeds
Olive oil spray
¼ cup chopped fresh chives, for garnish

Caramelized Onion
1 large or 2 small onions
Olive oil spray

In a bowl large enough to hold the tuna, whisk together the lime juice, sesame oil, salt, and pepper. Add the tuna and coat it well with the marinade. Cover and marinate in the refrigerator for 20 minutes.

To make the caramelized onion, after removing the outer layer of the onion, slice thin. Heat a nonstick frying pan over medium heat, coat it with olive oil spray, and add the onion. Cook for 15 minutes, stirring frequently to cook evenly, or until the onion is lightly browned.

Grind the sesame seeds in a coffee grinder and spread them on a plate. Remove the tuna from the marinade and dredge in the ground sesame, pressing the sesame into the tuna so it will stick. Dispose of the remaining marinade.

Heat an electric grill or grill pan over medium-high heat and coat with olive oil spray. Put the tuna on the grill and cook for 2 minutes each side, or until the tuna is pink in the center. Remove from the grill and plate with the caramelized onion. Garnish with chopped chives. Serves 2.

NUTRITION PER SERVING: 462 Calories | 44 g Protein | 15 g Carbohydrates | 25 g Fat

CHICKEN AND PEPPERS

STAGE 3

1 tablespoon extra virgin olive oil

1 cup sliced onions

2 garlic cloves, chopped

¼ cup whole wheat flour or all-purpose flour

¼ teaspoon salt

Freshly ground black pepper

2 skinless, boneless chicken breasts or 4 thighs

2 red or yellow bell peppers, sliced

½ cup chopped fresh parsley

Heat a large pot and coat it with the extra virgin olive oil. Add the onions and garlic and cook for 3 to 4 minutes over medium heat. Spread the flour on a plate and season with salt and pepper. Dredge the chicken in the seasoned flour to coat well. Move the onions to the sides of the pot and place the chicken in the bottom. Cook over medium heat for 5 minutes, or until the chicken is slightly browned. Add the peppers, parsley, and 1 cup water. Bring to a boil, then lower the heat and simmer, covered, for 30 minutes, or until the chicken is cooked through. Plate 1 breast of chicken or 2 thighs with half of the peppers and onions and spoon the sauce from the pot over the chicken. Serves 2.

NUTRITION PER SERVING: 321 Calories | 32 g Protein | 29 g Carbohydrates | 9 g Fat

CHICKEN QUESADILLAS WITH TOMATO SALSA

Tomato Salsa

1 tomato, chopped

1 yellow bell pepper, finely chopped

¼ cup finely chopped cilantro

Juice of ½ lime

Freshly ground black pepper

Chicken Quesadillas

10 ounces cooked skinless, boneless chicken breast, cut into strips

½ cup finely chopped fresh cilantro

¼ cup finely chopped scallions

½ cup shredded low-fat cheese: Cheddar, Monterey Jack, or American

2 whole wheat tortillas

Shake of cumin

Shake of turmeric

¼ teaspoon salt

Freshly ground black pepper

Olive oil spray

¼ cup nonfat plain yogurt

To make the salsa, gently mix the tomato, yellow pepper, and cilantro. Add the lime juice and black pepper.

To make one quesadilla, spread half of the chicken, cilantro, scallions, and cheese evenly across one half of a tortilla. Sprinkle with cumin, turmeric, salt, and pepper, then fold the other side of the tortilla over to form a half circle. Heat a nonstick frying pan over medium heat and coat with olive oil spray. Place the filled tortilla in the pan and cook on each side for 2 to 3 minutes, until golden brown. Repeat the steps to make the second quesadilla. Plate with yogurt and salsa on the side. Serves 2.

NUTRITION PER SERVING: 385 Calories | 47 g Protein | 34 g Carbohydrates | 7 g Fat

MINESTRONE RUSTICA

Olive oil spray

1 cup finely chopped onions

1 cup finely chopped celery

1 cup finely chopped carrots

4 garlic cloves, minced

One 15-ounce can diced or crushed tomatoes

One 15-ounce can cannellini or kidney beans, drained and rinsed

½ cup chopped fresh parsley

1 potato, finely diced

1 sprig fresh rosemary

¼ teaspoon salt

Freshly ground black pepper

3 cups baby spinach

2 teaspoons grated Parmesan cheese or other hard cheese, for garnish

Heat a large pot and coat it with olive oil spray. Add the onions, celery, carrots, and garlic and cook for 10 minutes over medium heat. Put the tomatoes, beans, parsley, potato, rosemary, and 4 cups water into the pot. Season with salt and pepper. Bring to a boil, then turn the heat down and simmer for 15 minutes. Add the spinach, stir well, and simmer for 10 minutes more. When done, remove the rosemary stem; the leaves will have fallen off and flavored the soup. Serve in bowls with a sprinkle of Parmesan. Serves 3.

NUTRITION PER SERVING: 271 Calories | 12 g Protein | 54 g Carbohydrates | 2 g Fat

SHRIMP SCAMPI WITH LINGUINE

Shrimp, garlic, and olive oil are a classic combination. This dish gets its bright, fresh flavor from healthy ingredients like fresh parsley and zesty lemon.

1 tablespoon extra virgin olive oil

3 garlic cloves, crushed

8 large or 10 medium shrimp, peeled and deveined

¼ teaspoon salt

Freshly ground black pepper

Juice of 1 lemon

½ cup finely chopped fresh parsley

½ pound whole wheat linguine or spaghetti

Heat a nonstick skillet over medium heat. Add the extra virgin olive oil and garlic and sauté for 2 minutes. Add the shrimp, season with salt and pepper, and cook over medium heat for 4 to 5 minutes, turning once, until the shrimp are pink. Remove from the heat and add the lemon juice and parsley.

While the shrimp are cooking, cook the linguine. Fill a large pot halfway with cold water and bring to a boil. When the water boils, add the pasta and cook over high heat for 7 to 8 minutes or according to directions on package. Test the pasta and remove when al dente, or soft enough to eat but still firm. Drain the pasta well, then toss with the shrimp and coat well with the sauce. Serves 2.

NUTRITION PER SERVING: 495 Calories | 21 g Protein | 90 g Carbohydrates | 10 g Fat

CHICKEN CURRY

STAGE

1 tablespoon extra virgin olive oil

½ cup chopped onion

3 garlic cloves, minced

2 teaspoons peeled, minced fresh ginger

½ cup canned crushed tomatoes

½ teaspoon turmeric

½ teaspoon cumin

½ teaspoon cardamom

¼ teaspoon salt

Freshly ground black pepper

1 pound skinless, boneless chicken breasts

Olive oil spray

3 tablespoons whole wheat flour or all-purpose flour

¼ cup chopped fresh parsley

To make the curry sauce, heat a large pot with a lid and coat it with the extra virgin olive oil. Add the onion, garlic, and ginger and sauté for 5 minutes over medium heat, stirring occasionally. Add the crushed tomatoes and 1½ cups water. Turn the heat off. Mix in the turmeric, cumin, cardamom, salt, and pepper. These spices give the sauce the distinctive curry color and flavor.

Before adding the chicken to the curry, brown it separately for added flavor. Heat a nonstick frying pan and coat it with olive oil spray. Cut the chicken into 1-inch cubes. Spread the flour across a plate and dredge the chicken in the flour to coat well. Place the chicken in the pan and cook for 5 minutes over medium heat, turning, or until slightly browned on all sides. Place the chicken in the pot with the curry sauce and coat well. Stir in the parsley. Cover the pot and bring to a boil, then lower the heat and simmer for 20 minutes. Serve the chicken and sauce over brown rice. Serves 2.

NUTRITION PER SERVING: 396 Calories | 55 g Protein | 17 g Carbohydrates | 11 g Fat

VEGETARIAN CURRY

1 tablespoon extra virgin olive oil

½ cup chopped onion

3 garlic cloves, minced

2 teaspoons minced ginger

½ cup canned crushed tomatoes

½ teaspoon turmeric

½ teaspoon cumin

½ teaspoon cardamom

¼ teaspoon salt

Freshly ground black pepper

4 cups cauliflower florets

1 cup canned kidney beans or garbanzo beans (chickpeas),
   drained and rinsed

½ cup frozen peas, thawed

¼ cup chopped fresh parsley

To make the curry sauce, heat a large pot with a lid and coat with the extra virgin olive oil. Add the onion, garlic, and ginger and sauté for 5 minutes over medium heat, stirring occasionally. Add the crushed tomatoes and 1½ cups water. Turn the heat off. Mix in the turmeric, cumin, cardamom, salt, and pepper. These spices give the sauce the distinctive curry color and flavor.

Put the cauliflower, beans, and peas in the pot and coat with the curry sauce. Cover and simmer for 7 to 8 minutes, until the cauliflower is fork-tender. Stir in the parsley. Serve the vegetables, beans, and sauce over brown rice. Serves 2.

NUTRITION PER SERVING: 286 Calories | 14 g Protein | 44 g Carbohydrates | 8 g Fat

Soups and Sides

SPINACH LEEK SOUP

2½ cups peeled, chopped potatoes (3 medium potatoes)

Two 10-ounce packages frozen spinach

½ cup finely chopped leek, white and light green parts only, rinsed
   thoroughly

3 garlic cloves, minced

½ teaspoon salt

Freshly ground black pepper

¼ teaspoon cumin

¼ teaspoon turmeric

Place the potatoes in a pot and cover with water. Bring to a boil and simmer for 8 to 10 minutes, until the potatoes are fork-tender. Transfer the potatoes to a strainer and let drain.

Meanwhile, put 5 cups water and the frozen spinach in a large pot with a lid. Defrost the spinach over medium-high heat. When the spinach is soft, add the cooked potatoes, leek, garlic, salt, and pepper. Cover the pot and simmer over medium heat for 12 minutes. Remove from the heat, let the soup cool, then transfer the soup to a blender and blend until smooth. Return the soup to the pot, season with cumin and turmeric, stir well, and heat through. Serves 5.

NUTRITION PER SERVING: 74 Calories | 5 g Protein | 14 g Carbohydrates | 1 g Fat

OVEN-ROASTED ROSEMARY POTATOES

Roasted in the oven, the potatoes get nice and brown and the garlic caramelizes.

STAGE 3

    2 potatoes, peeled and diced
    2 garlic cloves, sliced
    1 tablespoon chopped fresh or ½ teaspoon dried rosemary
    ¼ teaspoon salt
    Freshly ground black pepper
    Olive oil spray

Preheat an oven or toaster oven to 375°F. Spread the potatoes on a baking pan and sprinkle with the garlic, rosemary, salt, and pepper. Mist with olive oil spray and bake until fork-tender and golden brown, 15 to 20 minutes, turning them once midway through baking. Serves 2.

NUTRITION PER SERVING: 189 Calories | 4 g Protein | 38 g Carbohydrates | 3 g Fat

CORN AND TOMATO SALSA

    1 cup steamed corn
    10 cherry or grape tomatoes, halved
    2 stalks scallions, chopped
    Juice of ½ lime
    ¼ teaspoon cumin
    Pinch of salt
    Freshly ground black pepper

Let the corn cool to room temperature and mix with the tomatoes and scallions. Combine the lime juice, cumin, salt, and pepper in a cup. Pour the mixture over the salsa and stir to coat well. Serves 2.

NUTRITION PER SERVING: 90 Calories | 3 g Protein | 20 g Carbohydrates | 1 g Fat

Desserts

POMEGRANATE BANANA PARFAIT

1 cup nonfat plain yogurt

1 banana, sliced

2 tablespoons unsweetened pomegranate juice

In a parfait or wine glass, layer the yogurt, banana, and pomegranate concentrate. Serves 1.

NUTRITION PER SERVING: 218 Calories | 11 g Protein | 50 g Carbohydrates | 0.39 g Fat

KIWI CRUNCH PARFAIT

1 cup nonfat plain yogurt

1 kiwi, peeled and sliced

2 teaspoons Omega Blast Granola (page 256)

In a parfait or wine glass, layer the yogurt, kiwi, and granola. Serves 1.

NUTRITION PER SERVING: 208 Calories | 16 g Protein | 33 g Carbohydrates | 2 g Fat

GRILLED PEACHES

The warm cooked fruit tastes like peach pie. For best results, use peaches that are a little soft and ripe.

Olive oil spray

2 ripe peaches, halved and pitted

Heat a grill pan or electric grill and coat with olive oil spray. Place the peach halves cut side down on the grill and cook on medium for 5 to 7 minutes, until brown char marks form on the peaches. Serves 2.

NUTRITION PER SERVING: 45 Calories | 1 g Protein | 10 g Carbohydrates | 0.58 g Fat

Stages 1, 2, and 3

Bonus Recipes

Readers following our meal plans and recipes have expressed their enthusiasm for the culinary creations in the Fat Resistance Diet. On many occasions they have told us, "We want more recipes!"

So we went back to the test kitchen, to the green market, to the farm stands and the supermarket. We picked and chopped fresh herbs and tomatoes. We made our favorite meals and wrote down each step.

Here are more than 25 exciting new recipes from our kitchen to yours, featuring more of the international flavors that we enjoy and want to share with you. Each recipe indicates the meal and the stage in which it can be used, so you have more variety than ever. Stage 1 recipes can be used in all three stages; Stage 2 recipes, in Stages 2 and 3; but Stage 3 recipes are for Stage 3 only. Enjoy!

Breakfasts

GREEK OMELET

STAGE 1

Olive oil spray

1 garlic clove, minced

3 egg whites, lightly beaten

Freshly ground black pepper

2 tablespoons crumbled feta cheese

1 cup chopped baby spinach

1 tomato, sliced

Heat a small nonstick frying pan. Coat the pan with olive oil spray, add the garlic, and cook for 1 to 2 minutes over medium heat. Pour the egg whites over the garlic and season with black pepper. Spread the feta cheese and spinach evenly over the eggs and cook for 4 minutes, or until the eggs are set. Fold one side of the omelet over the other to form a half circle and cook for 2 minutes more. Plate with tomato slices on the side. Serves 1.

NUTRITION PER SERVING: 146 Calories | 15 g Protein | 10 g Carbohydrates | 5 g Fat

FRESH GREENS OMELET

Olive oil spray
3 egg whites, lightly beaten
¼ teaspoon salt
Freshly ground black pepper
2 stalks scallions, chopped
1 cup arugula, chopped
½ cup fresh parsley, chopped
1 tomato, sliced

STAGE 1

Heat a small nonstick frying pan. Coat the pan with olive oil spray, add the egg whites, and season with salt and pepper. Cook for 1 to 2 minutes over medium heat. Spread the scallions, arugula, and parsley evenly over the eggs and cook for 4 to 5 minutes, or until the eggs are set. Fold one side of the omelet over the other to form a half circle and cook for 2 minutes more. Plate with tomato slices on the side. Serves 1.

NUTRITION PER SERVING: 105 Calories | 12 g Protein | 9 g Carbohydrates | 2 g Fat

SPANISH OMELET

Olive oil spray

⅓ cup finely diced red, yellow, or orange bell pepper

⅓ cup finely diced onion

3 egg whites, lightly beaten

¼ teaspoon salt

Freshly ground black pepper

⅓ cup diced tomato

¼ cup chopped fresh cilantro

2 cups mixed salad greens

Heat a small nonstick frying pan. Coat the pan with olive oil spray, add the pepper and onion, and cook for 3 to 5 minutes over medium heat. Pour the egg whites over the vegetables and season with salt and pepper. Spread the tomato and cilantro evenly over the eggs and cook for 4 minutes, or until the eggs are set. Fold one side of the omelet over the other to form a half circle and cook for 2 minutes more. Serve over a bed of mixed salad greens. Serves 1.

NUTRITION PER SERVING: 115 Calories | 12 g Protein | 9 g Carbohydrates | 2 g Fat

CHERRY GREEN SMOOTHIE

1 cup frozen pitted cherries

1 cup nonfat milk or unsweetened soymilk

1 scoop SlimGreens

1 tablespoon freshly ground flaxseeds

1 tablespoon whey protein concentrate or soy protein powder

Put the cherries and milk into a blender and blend until smooth. Add the SlimGreens, ground flaxseeds, and whey protein. Blend again. Pour into a tall glass and enjoy! Serves 1.

NUTRITION PER SERVING: 242 Calories | 15 g Protein | 35 g Carbohydrates | 4 g Fat

POMEGRANATE SMOOTHIE

STAGE

½ cup unsweetened pomegranate juice

1 cup ice

¾ cup nonfat milk or unsweetened soymilk

1 tablespoon freshly ground flaxseeds

1 tablespoon whey protein concentrate or soy protein powder

Put ice and pomegranate juice into a blender. Add the milk and blend. Add in the ground flaxseeds and whey protein. Blend until smooth. Pour into a tall glass and enjoy! Serves 1.

NUTRITION PER SERVING: 230 Calories | 13 g Protein | 35 g Carbohydrates | 4 g Fat

BERRY GREEN SMOOTHIE

1 cup frozen blueberries

1 cup nonfat milk or unsweetened soymilk

1 scoop SlimGreens

1 tablespoon freshly ground flaxseeds

1 tablespoon whey protein concentrate or soy protein powder

Put the blueberries and milk into a blender and blend until the berries have turned the milk a deep, rich blue. Add the SlimGreens, ground flaxseeds, and whey protein. Blend until smooth. Pour into a tall glass and enjoy! Serves 1.

NUTRITION PER SERVING: 242 Calories | 15 g Protein | 35 g Carbohydrates | 4 g Fat

Lunch

CAFÉ SALAD

4 cups salad greens

½ tomato, cut in wedges

2 carrots, shredded

1 bell pepper, sliced

1 red onion, sliced

1 cup canned garbanzo beans (chickpeas), drained and rinsed

2 teaspoons extra virgin olive oil

¼ teaspoon salt

Freshly ground black pepper

2 tablespoons freshly ground flaxseeds

½ avocado, sliced

½ cup fresh parsley, chopped

Place greens in a salad bowl. Add the tomato, carrots, bell pepper, onion, and garbanzo beans. Toss with the extra virgin olive oil, salt, pepper and flaxseeds. Top with avocado and sprinkle with parsley. Serves 2.

NUTRITION PER SERVING: 237 Calories | 9 g Protein | 24 g Carbohydrates | 15g Fat

GOAT CHEESE SALAD

STAGE 1

4 cups mixed greens

8 grape or cherry tomatoes

½ cup parsley, chopped

2 teaspoons Pesto Vinaigrette (page 229)

1 pear, thinly sliced

2 tablespoons low-fat goat cheese

1 tablespoon sliced almonds

Place the greens in a salad bowl. Add the tomatoes, parsley, and Pesto Vinaigrette and toss. Plate salad into two bowls. Divide the sliced pear, goat cheese, and almonds evenly and spread over the salads. Serves 2.

NUTRITION PER SERVING: 198 Calories | 9 g Protein | 24 g Carbohydrates | 9 g Fat

APPLE WALNUT SALAD

1 apple, peeled and sliced

Juice of ½ lemon

3 heads endive

½ yellow bell pepper, thinly sliced

8 walnut halves

Pinch of salt

Freshly ground black pepper

1 teaspoon Pomegranate Lime Dressing (page 227)

In a small bowl, coat the apple with lemon juice. In a large bowl, toss together the endive, bell pepper, and walnuts. Arrange the apples across the top of the salad. Season with salt and pepper. Dress with Pomegranate Lime Dressing just before serving. Serves 1.

NUTRITION PER SERVING: 232 Calories | 7 g Protein | 32 g Carbohydrates | 11 g Fat

SESAME SALAD

2 cups mixed salad greens

2 tablespoons fresh cilantro, chopped

2 cups broccoli, cut into very small florets

1 cup canned kidney beans, drained and rinsed

8 cherry or grape tomatoes, halved

Pinch of salt

Freshly ground black pepper

1 teaspoon toasted sesame oil

1 teaspoon freshly ground sesame seeds

STAGE 1

In a large bowl, toss together the salad greens, cilantro, broccoli, kidney beans, and tomatoes. Season with salt and pepper. Dress with sesame oil and a sprinkle of sesame seeds just before serving. Serves 2.

NUTRITION PER SERVING: 224 Calories | 13 g Protein | 37 g Carbohydrates | 4 g Fat

CAPRESE PANINI

⅓ cup low-fat mozzarella cheese

2 thin slices multigrain or whole wheat bread

½ tomato, sliced

4 basil leaves

Pinch of salt

Freshly ground black pepper

Place mozzarella on one slice of bread. Add the tomato, basil, salt, and pepper, then cover with the other slice of bread. Preheat an electric grill or panini press. Place the panini on the grill and close. Grill for 3 to 4 minutes, or until the cheese melts and the bread is nicely browned. Serves 1.

COOKING NOTE: When a grill is not available, use a nonstick frying pan. Preheat the pan on medium heat, place the panini into the pan, and press down with a spatula. Cook for 2 minutes, or until the cheese starts to melt, then flip over and cook for 2 more minutes, pressing down with spatula.

NUTRITION PER SERVING: 234 Calories | 17 g Protein | 28 g Carbohydrates | 7 g Fat

FRESH GUACAMOLE PANINI

¼ avocado, thinly sliced

Juice of ½ lime

3 slices red onion

½ tomato, sliced

2 thin slices multigrain or whole wheat bread

2 tablespoons fresh cilantro, chopped

Sprinkle of cumin

Pinch of salt

Freshly ground black pepper

In a small bowl, coat the avocado with lime juice. Spread the avocado, onion, and tomato over one slice of bread. Sprinkle with cilantro and cumin. Season with salt and pepper, then cover with the other slice of bread. Cut the panini in half and enjoy! Serves 1.

NUTRITION PER SERVING: 302 Calories | 8 g Protein | 47 g Carbohydrates | 11 g Fat

Dinner

ISLAND GRILLED SHRIMP

Juice of 1 lime

1 tablespoon extra virgin olive oil

2 cloves garlic, minced

¼ teaspoon salt

Freshly ground black pepper

½ pound medium or large shrimp, peeled and deveined

1 cup pineapple, cubed

3 stalks scallions, cut into 3-inch sticks

¼ cup fresh basil, chopped

2 teaspoons freshly ground sesame seeds

In a bowl, whisk together lime juice, extra virgin olive oil, garlic, salt, and pepper. Add the shrimp and coat well with the mixture. Cover the bowl and refrigerate for 20 minutes.

Heat an electric grill or grill pan. Remove the shrimp from the marinade and discard the marinade. Place the shrimp, pineapple, and scallions on the grill and cook for 4 to 5 minutes, turning once, or until the shrimp are pink.

Take the shrimp, pineapple, and scallions off the grill and arrange on a large plate. Sprinkle with basil and sesame seeds. Serve with one of our side dish recipes such as Swiss Chard (page 340) or Kale (page 341). For a summertime meal, pair the shrimp with Asian Coleslaw (page 231). Serves 2.

NUTRITION PER SERVING: 252 Calories | 24 g Protein | 15 g Carbohydrates | 10 g Fat

TRADITIONAL MISO SOUP WITH VEGETABLES

STAGE 1

2 cups bonito flakes

4 carrots, chopped

1 small daikon, peeled and sliced

1 onion, sliced

1 cup shiitake mushrooms, sliced

7 ounces tofu, cut into small cubes

1 package baby spinach

2 tablespoons wakame

4½ tablespoons miso paste

2 stalks scallions, cut diagonally into 2-inch pieces

Bring 8 cups water to a boil. Add the bonito flakes and turn off the heat. Let stand for 10 minutes. This creates a "dashi" stock. Remove bonito flakes from dashi stock with a strainer. Discard the bonito flakes.

Bring stock to a simmer over moderate heat and add the carrots and daikon. Cook for 2 minutes. Add the onion, mushrooms, tofu, spinach, and wakame and cook for 5 minutes. Turn off the heat. Stir in the miso paste. Add scallions on top of the soup. Ladle 2 cups in each of four bowls. Serves 4.

SHOPPING NOTES: Miso paste, made from soybeans, is high in protein and a good source of trace minerals. A traditional staple of the Japanese kitchen, miso paste is so versatile, it is now used by American chefs. Fresh miso is becoming more widely available in supermarkets, health-food stores, and Asian markets. Look for it in the refrigerated section.

Two American producers of miso are South River Miso Company in Massachusetts (www.southrivermiso.com) and Great Eastern Sun in North Carolina (www.great-eastern-sun.com). For bonito flakes, check the Japanese-ingredient section at your health-food store. You can also order bonito flakes online from Eden foods, which carries a wide variety of Japanese foods, at www.edenfoods.com.

NUTRITION PER SERVING: 142 Calories | 11 g Protein | 20 g Carbohydrates | 4 g Fat

SASHIMI STYLE SALAD

STAGE 1

4 cups mixed greens

1 orange, peeled and cut into slices

3 stalks scallions, chopped

¼ cup chopped fresh parsley

Juice of 1 lime

½ teaspoon toasted sesame oil

4 ounces smoked salmon, cut into slices

¼ avocado, sliced

Dash of salt

Freshly ground black pepper

1 sheet nori seaweed, torn into small pieces

1 teaspoon freshly ground sesame seeds

In a large bowl, mix the greens, orange, scallions, and parsley with lime juice and sesame oil. Divide evenly between two bowls. Place the salmon and avocado on top of the salad. Season with salt and pepper. Finish by sprinkling the salad with nori and sesame seeds. Serves 2.

SHOPPING NOTE: For nori, check the Japanese-ingredient section at your health-food store. You can also order nori online from Eden foods, which carries a wide variety of Japanese foods, at www.edenfoods.com.

NUTRITION PER SERVING: 258 Calories | 25 g Protein | 19 g Carbohydrates | 9 g Fat

SOBA NOODLES WITH DASHI

2 pieces kombu seaweed

4 cups bonito flakes

4 carrots, chopped

1 cup shiitake mushrooms, sliced

1 package baby spinach

2 tablespoons ginger, minced

8 ounces soba noodles

3 stalks scallions, cut diagonally into 2-inch pieces

2 tablespoons soy sauce

To make the dashi broth, bring 10 cups water to a boil in a large stockpot. Add the kombu and boil for 3 minutes. Add the bonito flakes and simmer for 3 minutes, then turn off the heat. Let stand for 10 minutes. Remove kombu and bonito flakes with a strainer and discard.

Bring dashi broth to a simmer over moderate heat, add the carrots, and cook for 2 minutes. Add the mushrooms and spinach and cook for 5 minutes.

To cook the soba noodles, fill another stockpot ⅔ with water and bring to a boil. Place soba noodles into the boiling water and boil for 3 to 4 minutes, or according to directions on the package. Test the soba and remove when al dente, or soft enough to eat but still firm. Remove and place in strainer and rinse with cold water.

Plate soba into four bowls, add dashi broth with vegetables, and top with scallions and season with soy sauce, if desired. Serves 4.

SHOPPING NOTE: For kombu, bonito flakes, and soba noodles, check the Japanese-ingredient section at your health-food store. You can also order these ingredients online from Eden foods, which carries a wide variety of Japanese foods, at www.edenfoods.com.

NUTRITION PER SERVING: 252 Calories | 11 g Protein | 45 g Carbohydrates | 1 g Fat

GINGER BROCCOLI STIR-FRY

1 teaspoon extra virgin olive oil

½ cup peeled, julienned fresh ginger

4 cloves fresh garlic, chopped

1 onion, sliced

1 cup daikon, peeled and chopped

4 stalks celery, chopped

4 cups broccoli, cut into florets

7 ounces firm or extra firm tofu

1 cup whole wheat linguine or spaghetti, cooked

1 tablespoon miso

¼ teaspoon turmeric

½ cup chopped parsley

Heat a large skillet on medium heat and coat with the extra virgin olive oil. Add the ginger, garlic, onion, daikon, and celery to the pan and sauté for 4 minutes, stirring frequently. Add ½ cup water, broccoli, and tofu. Cover and cook for 4 minutes, or until the broccoli is fork-tender. Remove cover, add the linguine, and toss with the vegetables. Stir in the miso and turmeric. Sprinkle with parsley. Serves 2.

NUTRITION PER SERVING: 304 Calories | 14 g Protein | 56 g Carbohydrates | 5 g Fat

Side Vegetable

MUSHROOMS, PEPPERS, ZUCCHINI, ONIONS, AND GARLIC

1 teaspoon extra virgin olive oil

1 cup shiitake mushrooms, sliced

4 cloves garlic, chopped

1 onion, thinly sliced

2 zucchini, thinly sliced

1 bell pepper, thinly sliced

¼ teaspoon salt

Freshly ground black pepper

½ cup basil, chopped

STAGE 1

Heat a frying pan over medium heat and coat it with the extra virgin olive oil. Add the mushrooms and sauté on medium heat for 10 minutes, turning frequently, or until slightly caramelized. Remove the mushrooms to a bowl.

Add the garlic, onion, zucchini, and bell pepper to the pan and season with salt and black pepper. Sauté on medium heat, turning frequently, for 5 minutes. Put the mushrooms into the pan and toss together with the vegetables. Sprinkle with basil to serve. Serves 2.

NUTRITION PER SERVING: 143 Calories | 5 g Protein | 28 g Carbohydrates | 3 g Fat

SWISS CHARD

1 bunch Swiss chard, chopped (yields 3 cups cooked)

1 teaspoon extra virgin olive oil

2 cloves of garlic

¼ teaspoon salt

Freshly ground black pepper

Prepare the Swiss chard by folding large leaves together, stem side out. With scissors, cut large stems from leaves, or you may pull leaves from stems. Give the leaves a very good rinse, then spin in a salad spinner, and repeat rinse-and-spin. Give leaves a good chop. Heat a large skillet and add the extra virgin olive oil and garlic. Add the Swiss chard and ½ cup water to the pan, cover, and steam, stirring occasionally, for 5 to 7 minutes, or until tender. Season with salt and pepper. Serves 2.

GARDENING TIP: If you plant a vegetable garden, plan to grow Swiss chard. It will reward you with tender young leaves, which you should pick, and more will grow. When leaves are tender, you may wish to chop the stems as well as the leaves. We enjoyed our Swiss chard so much that this year we grew extra in large clay pots.

NUTRITION PER SERVING: 79 Calories | 5 g Protein | 12 g Carbohydrates | 2 g Fat

KALE

1 bunch kale
1 teaspoon extra virgin olive oil
4 cloves garlic, chopped
¼ teaspoon salt
Freshly ground black pepper
Juice of ½ lemon

STAGE 1

Prepare kale by removing the stems and tearing them into pieces. Give the leaves a good rinse, spin in a salad spinner, and repeat rinse-and-spin. Chop leaves well. Heat a large skillet on medium heat and add the extra virgin olive oil. Add the garlic and sauté for 2 minutes. Add the kale and ½ cup water. Cover and steam, stirring occasionally, for 10 to 15 minutes, or until leaves are tender. Toss with salt and pepper. Finish with a squeeze of lemon. Serves 4.

GARDENING TIP: Kale is a very hearty plant to grow in your garden. Our kale had edible leaves throughout the winter, producing a beautiful 3-foot-tall plant with lovely yellow flowers in the spring.

NUTRITION PER SERVING: 75 Calories | 4 g Protein | 13 g Carbohydrates | 2 g Fat

SESAME SPINACH

1 teaspoon toasted sesame oil

3 cloves garlic, chopped

1 package baby spinach

1 teaspoon soy sauce

1 tablespoon freshly ground sesame seeds

Heat a nonstick skillet over medium heat and add the sesame oil. Add the garlic and spinach and sauté, stirring frequently, for 3 or 4 minutes, or until the spinach wilts. Turn off the heat, add the soy sauce, and sprinkle with sesame seeds. Serves 2.

NUTRITION PER SERVING: 65 Calories | 3 g Protein | 4 g Carbohydrates | 4 g Fat

BRUSSELS SPROUTS

2 cups Brussels sprouts (1 pint)

2 cloves garlic

¼ teaspoon salt

1 teaspoon olive oil

Freshly ground black pepper

Trim the stems of the Brussels sprouts, then cut in half. Bring an inch of water to a boil in a saucepan. Add the Brussels sprouts, garlic, and salt. Cover and steam for 7 to 8 minutes, or until fork-tender. Drain the water.

Heat a frying pan on medium heat, then coat with the olive oil. Add the Brussels sprouts to the pan and sauté, stirring often, for 2 to 3 minutes, or until slightly browned. Season with pepper. Serves 2.

NUTRITION PER SERVING: 81 Calories | 4 g Protein | 12 g Carbohydrates | 2 g Fat

Dessert

CHERRIES IN THE SNOW

½ cup nonfat ricotta cheese
1 cup pitted frozen or fresh cherries
1 teaspoon cherry concentrate

Spoon the ricotta into a dessert dish and arrange the cherries on top. Drizzle with cherry concentrate. Serves 1.

NUTRITION PER SERVING: 206 Calories | 12 g Protein | 33 g Carbohydrates | 1 g Fat

CINNAMON APPLE DELIGHT

½ cup nonfat ricotta cheese
1 apple, peeled and sliced
1 teaspoon cinnamon
8 walnut halves, chopped

Spoon the ricotta into a dessert dish. Using another small bowl, dredge the apple slices in the cinnamon and coat well. Arrange the apple slices on the ricotta and sprinkle with walnuts. Serves 1.

NUTRITION PER SERVING: 294 Calories | 12 g Protein | 36 g Carbohydrates | 10 g Fat

TROPICAL FRUIT SALAD

2 cups cubed pineapple

1 cup organic seedless red grapes

1 kiwi, peeled and sliced

1 banana, peeled and sliced

Juice of ½ lemon

5 mint leaves, chopped

STAGE 1

In a large bowl, mix together the pineapple, grapes, kiwi, and banana slices. Sprinkle with fresh-squeezed lemon juice and mint leaves. Serves 2.

NUTRITION PER SERVING: 208 Calories | 2 g Protein | 54 g Carbohydrates | 1 g Fat

PEACH SPICE DELIGHT

½ cup nonfat ricotta cheese

½ teaspoon cinnamon

1 peach, peeled, pitted, and sliced

1 teaspoon sliced almonds

In a small bowl, stir together the ricotta and cinnamon. Spoon into a dessert dish and arrange peach slices on top. Sprinkle with sliced almonds. Serves 1.

NUTRITION PER SERVING: 154 Calories | 11 g Protein | 20 g Carbohydrates | 1 g Fat

appendix

~~~

Stage 1 Shopping Lists

Almost everything you need to follow the Fat Resistance Diet should be on the shelves of your local supermarket or health food store, so you can follow the diet plan one day at a time. I recommend that you shop frequently and buy your food as fresh as possible. To help you stock your pantry, I created a list of everything you'll need to complete Stage 1 exactly as I have laid it out in Part Three. You'll notice that certain foods are marked with an asterisk (*). Try to purchase these foods as close to the day of actual consumption as possible, as they can rapidly lose freshness and nutritional value.

In Your Pantry

On the following pages is a list of pantry and refrigerator staples that you will need on the Fat Resistance Diet.

CANNED/FROZEN PRODUCE/JUICES

Black beans, 15-ounce can
Blueberries, frozen, two 10-ounce packages
Blueberry concentrate, 6 ounces
Capers, one 3-ounce jar
Cherry concentrate, 6 ounces
Garbanzo beans (chickpeas), 15-ounce can
Green peas, frozen, one 10-ounce package
Pineapple chunks in their own juice (not syrup), 15-ounce can
Pomegranate juice, 32 ounces
Strawberries, frozen, one 10-ounce package
Tomatoes, crushed, 15-ounce can
Vegetable juice, 2 quarts

MEAT/PROTEIN

Tuna, water-packed, two 6-ounce cans

NUTS/GRAINS

Almond butter
Almonds, 1 pound
Flaxseeds, 1 pound
Sesame seeds, 4 ounces
Walnut halves, 1 pound

Spices/Condiments/Oils

Cardamom, ground
Cinnamon, ground
Cloves, whole

Cumin, ground
Dill (optional)
Five-spice powder
Garlic powder
Ginger, fresh and/or ground
Lemongrass powder (optional)
Olive oil, extra virgin (olive oil spray or mister—optional)
Onion, dried
Peppercorns, black
Rosemary, fresh or dried
Thyme, fresh or dried
Turmeric
Salt
Sesame oil, toasted
Soy sauce, low-sodium
Vinegar
Walnut oil

Miscellaneous

Cocoa powder, unsweetened
Coffee, instant (if desired for Iced Mocha Latte)
Coffee beans, regular or decaffeinated (if desired)
Tea, green, 20 bags
Tea, green, loose, small amount
Whey protein concentrate, 1 pound

Week 1 Shopping List

PRODUCE

Apples, 4
*Arugula, 2 bunches
*Asparagus, 1 pound
Avocado, 1
Bananas, 2
*Basil, 2 bunches
Broccoli, 2 bunches
*Cabbage, green, 1 head
Carrots, 2 pounds
Celery, 2 large bunches
Chives, 1 bunch
*Cilantro, 1 bunch
Cucumbers, 3
Eggplant, 1 small, 8 ounces
*Endive, Belgian, 1 head (optional)
Garlic, fresh, several heads
Ginger, fresh and/or ground
Grapefruit, 3
Green beans, 1 pound
*Greens, mixed salad, 8-ounce bag
Leeks, 1 bunch
Lemons, 6
Limes, 6
Mango, 1
Mint, 1 bunch
*Mushrooms, portobello, 2
Mushrooms, shiitake, 4 ounces
Onions, 11
Oranges, 3
Parsley, 2 bunches
Pears, 2

Peppers, bell, red or yellow, 6
*Romaine lettuce, 2 heads
Scallions, 2 bunches
*Spinach, baby, 8 ounces
Tomatoes, 20
Tomatoes, cherry or grape, 1 pint
Tomatoes, plum, 4

DAIRY

Cheddar or Monterey Jack cheese, low-fat, 2 ounces
Cottage cheese, low-fat, 8 ounces
Feta cheese, 4 ounces
Milk, low-fat/nonfat (as desired, for coffee)
Mozzarella cheese, shredded low-fat, 8 ounces
Parmesan cheese, 4 ounces
Ricotta cheese, nonfat, 15 ounces
Soymilk, unsweetened (as desired)
Yogurt, nonfat plain, 2 quarts

MEAT/PROTEIN

Chicken breasts, boneless and skinless, 1 pound
Eggs, 1½ dozen
*Fish fillets: flounder, sole, or tilapia, 2 pounds
Salmon, smoked, 8 ounces
Sirloin steak, 12 ounces
Tofu, firm or extra-firm, reduced-fat, 14 ounces
*Turkey, roasted, sliced, 4 ounces

Week 2 Shopping List

PRODUCE

Apples, 2
*Arugula, 2 bunches
Avocado, 1
Bananas, 2
*Basil, 2 bunches
Broccoli, 2 bunches
*Cabbage, 1 head (bok choy, Napa, or green)
Cantaloupe, 1
Carrots, 2 pounds
Celery, 2 bunches
Cherries, 4 ounces
Chives, 1 bunch
*Cilantro, 1 bunch
Cucumbers, 3
*Endive, Belgian, 1 head
Grapefruit, 4
*Greens, mixed salad, 8-ounce bag
Leeks, 1 bunch
Lemons, 4
Limes, 6
Mint, 1 bunch
Mushrooms, white button or shiitake, 4 ounces
Onions, red, 12
Onion, sweet 1
Oranges, 3
Parsley, 2 bunches
Pears, 2
Peppers, bell, red or yellow, 6
*Romaine lettuce, 1 head
Scallions, 1 bunch
*Spinach, baby, 8 ounces

Tomatoes, 3
Tomatoes, cherry or grape, 1 pint

DAIRY

Cottage cheese, low-fat, 8 ounces
Feta cheese, 4 ounces
Mozzarella cheese, shredded low-fat, 8 ounces
Ricotta cheese, nonfat, 15 ounces
Yogurt, nonfat plain, 1 quart

MEAT/PROTEIN

*Chicken breasts, boneless and skinless, 2 pounds
Eggs, 1½ dozen
*Fish fillets: flounder, sole, or tilapia, 1 pound
*Flank steak, 8 ounces
Salmon, smoked, 8 ounces
*Sea scallops, 1 pound
Shrimp, large, 8 ounces
Tofu, firm or extra-firm, 21 ounces

Resources

The Official Fat Resistance Diet Web site:
www.fatresistancediet.com

Our official Web site is the best place for information and products to help you achieve your weight-loss and health goals. SlimGreens, multivitamins, and other selected nutritional supplements can be ordered directly from our site. Sign up now for our newsletter to receive the latest articles, updates, links, and events. The site features Christina Galland's beautiful food photos, which illustrate the freshness, flavor, and fun that the diet is all about. Enjoy!

Air Purifiers
AllerAir Industries
888-852-8247
www.allerair.com
Aprilaire
800-334-6011
www.aprilaire.com
Bionaire
The Holmes Group
23B Spur Drive
El Paso, TX 79906
800-788-5350
www.bionaire.com

Beans
Eden Foods
701 Tecumseh Road
Clinton, Michigan 49236
888-424-3336
www.edenfoods.com

Westbrae Natural
The Hain Celestial Group
4600 Sleepytime Drive
Boulder, CO 80301
800-434-4246
www.westbrae.com

Canned Tomatoes
Muir Glen
General Mills
PO Box 9452
Minneapolis, MN 55440
800-624-4123
www.muirglen.com

Cherry Concentrate and Blueberry Concentrate
R.W. Knudsen
1 Strawberry Lane
Orrville, OH 44667-0280
www.knudsenjuices.com

Tree of Life
405 Golfway West Drive
St. Augustine, FL 32095
904-940-2100
www.treeoflife.com

Cleaning Products
Earth Friendly Products
44 Green Bay Road
Winnetka, Il 60093
800-335-3267
www.ecos.com
Ecover
PO Box 911058
Commerce, CA 90091
800-449-4925
www.ecover.com
Seventh Generation
60 Lake Street
Burlington, VT 05401
800-456-1191
www.seventhgeneration.com
Sun & Earth
221 King Manor Drive
King of Prussia, PA 19406
800-298-7861
www.sunandearth.com
Vermont Soap.com
616 Exchange Street
Middlebury, VT 05753
866-762-7482
www.vermontsoap.com

Coffee
Cafe Altura
760 East Santa Maria Street
Santa Paula, CA 93060
800-526-8328
www.cafealtura.com
Dean's Beans
50 Moore Avenue
Orange, MA 01364
800-325-3008
www.deansbeans.com

Green Mountain Coffee Roasters
33 Coffee Lane
Waterbury, VT 05676
888-879-4627
www.greenmountaincoffee.com
Jim's Organic Coffee
21 Patterson Brook Road
West Wareham, MA 02576
866-546-7674
www.jimsorganiccoffee.com
Organic Coffee Company
1933 Davis Street, Suite 308
San Leandro, CA 94577
800-829-1300
www.organiccoffeecompany.com
Veritas Organic Coffee
PO Box 8187
Bend, OR 97708
866-387-6927
www.veritascoffee.com

Eggs
Egg Innovations
3420 Highway West
Port Washington, WI 53074
800-337-1951
www.egginnovations.com
Pete and Gerry's Organic Eggs
140 Buffum Road
Monroe, NH 03771
800-GET-EGGS
www.peteandgerrys.com
Sauder's Eggs
570 Furnace Hills Pike
Lititz, PA 17543
800-233-0413
www.saudereggs.com

Frozen Vegetables
Cascadian Farms
General Mills
PO Box 9452
Minneapolis, MN 55440
800-624-4123
www.cascadianfarm.com

Furniture

Atlantic Adirondack Co.
2257 Vista Parkway, #23
West Palm Beach, FL 33411
866-869-8122
www.atlantic-adirondack.com

Green Culture
32 Rancho Circle
Lake Forest, CA 92630
877-204-7336
www.greenculture.com

Green Home
850 24th Avenue
San Francisco, CA 94121
877-282-6400
www.greenhome.com

Gardening

Clean Air Gardening
2266 Monitor Street
Dallas, TX 75207
214-819-9500
www.cleanairgardening.com

Extremely Green Gardening Company
PO Box 2021
Abington, MA 02351
781-878-5397
www.extremelygreen.com

Gardener's Supply Company
128 Intervale Road
Burlington, VT 05401
888-833-1412
www.gardeners.com

Gardens Alive!
5100 Schenley Place
Lawrenceburg, IN 47025
513-354-1482
www.gardensalive.com

Heirloom Seeds
PO Box 245
West Elizabeth, PA 15088
412-384-0852
www.heirloomseeds.com

The Natural Gardening Company
PO Box 750776
Petaluma CA 94975-0776
707-766-9303
www.naturalgardening.com

P. Allen Smith
www.pallensmith.com

Peaceful Valley Farm and Garden Supply
PO Box 2209
125 Clydesdale Court
Grass Valley, CA 95945
888-784-1722
www.groworganic.com

Planet Natural
1612 Gold Avenue
Bozeman, MT 59715
800-289-6656
www.planetnatural.com

Grains

Arrowhead Mills
The Hain Celestial Group
4600 Sleepytime Drive
Boulder, CO 80301
800-434-4246
www.arrowheadmills.com

Groceries

Whole Foods Market
512-477-4455
www.wholefoods.com

Home Improvement

AFM Safecoat
800-239-0321
www.afmsafecoat.com

Eco-Products
3655 Frontier Avenue
Boulder, CO 80301
303-449-1876
www.ecoproducts.com

EcoTimber
1611 Fourth Street
San Rafael, CA 94901
415-258-8454
www.ecotimber.com

Eco-Wares, Inc.
7634-B Progress Circle
West Melbourne, FL 32904
866-874-8070
www.eco-wares.com

The Environmental Home Center
4121 1st Avenue South
Seattle, WA 98134
800-281-9785
www.environmentalhomecenter.com

Forest Stewardship Council-U.S.
1155 30th Street NW, Suite 300
Washington, DC 20007
202-342-0413
www.fscus.org

Healthy Building Network
Institute for Local Self-Reliance
927 15th Street NW, 4th Floor
Washington, DC 20005
202-898-1610
www.healthybuilding.net

Nature's Carpet
494 Railway Street
Vancouver, BC V6A 1B1
Canada
800.667.5001
www.naturescarpet.com

Nature's Odor & Germ Control, Inc.
1521 North Jantzen Avenue, # 135
Portland, OR 97217-8100
888-884-6367
www.nogc.com

The Old Fashioned Milk Paint Company, Inc.
436 Main Street
Groton, MA 01450
866-350-6455
www.milkpaint.com

Tried & True Wood Finishes
14 Prospect Street
Trumansburg, NY 14886
607-387-9280
www.triedandtruewoodfinish.com

Linens and Bedding

A Natural Home
109 North Main Street
Fredericktown, OH 43019
866-239-4142
www.anaturalhome.com

EcoChoices
PO Box 1491
Glendora, CA 91740
626-969-3707
www.ecochoices.com

Gaiam
360 Interlocken Boulevard
Suite 300
Broomfield, CO 80021
877-989-6321
www.gaiam.com

Heart of Vermont
PO Box 612
Barre, VT 05641
800-639-4123
www.heartofvermont.com

Lifekind Products, Inc.
PO Box 1774
Grass Valley, CA 95945
800-284-4983
www.lifekind.com

Sachi Organics
523 West Cordova Road
Santa Fe, NM 87505
877-997-2244
www.sachiorganics.com

Magazines
Body + Soul
www.marthastewart.com/bodyandsoulmag
Fitness
www.fitnessmagazine.com

Men's Health
www.menshealth.com
Organic Gardening
www.organicgardening.com
Prevention
www.prevention.com
Women's Health
www.womenshealthmag.com

Natural Oils
Spectrum Organic Products
5341 Old Redwood Highway, Suite 400
Petaluma, CA 94954
www.spectrumorganics.com

Nonfat Plain Yogurt and Cheese
Horizon Organic
PO Box 17577
Boulder, CO 80308
888-494-3020
www.horizonorganic.com
Stonyfield Farm
10 Burton Drive
Londonderry, NH 03053
800-776-2697
www.stonyfield.com

Nutritional Software
Applied Nutrition
www.nutritionworkshop.com

Office Supplies
Dolphin Blue
1920 Abrams Parkway
Dallas, TX 75214-6218
800-932-7715
www.dolphinblue.com
Ecopaper.com
1860 Eastman Avenue, Suite 101
Ventura, CA 93003
805-444-4462
www.ecopaper.com
Green Earth Office Supply
PO Box 719
Redwood Estates, CA 95044

800-327-8449
www.greenearthofficesupply.com
Living Tree Paper Company
1430 Willamette Street, Suite 367
Eugene, OR 97401
800-309-2974
www.livingtreepaper.com
New Leaf Paper
116 New Montgomery Street, Suite
830
San Francisco, CA 94105
888-989-5323
www.newleafpaper.com

Organic Foods
Diamond Organics
1272 Highway 1
Moss Landing, CA 95039
888-674-2642
www.diamondorganics.com
Organic Valley Family of Farms
CROPP Cooperative
1 Organic Way
LaFarge, WI 54639
888-444-6455
www.organicvalley.coop

Personal Care
Avalon Natural Products
1105 Industrial Avenue
Petaluma, CA 94952
800-227-5120
www.avalonnaturalproducts.com
Dr. Hauschka Skincare Inc.
59 North Street
Hatfield, MA 01038
800-247-9907
www.drhauschka.com
Kiss My Face
PO Box 224
144 Main Street
Gardiner, NY 12525
800-404-1260
www.kissmyface.com

NatraCare
14901 East Hampden Avenue, Suite 190
Aurora, CO 80014
303-617-3476
www.naturacare.com
NEEDS, Inc.
800-634-1380
www.needs.com
Tom's of Maine
302 Lafayette Center
Kennebunk, ME 04043
800-367-8667
www.tomsofmaine.com
Weleda North America, Inc.
1 Closter Road
PO Box 675
Palisades, NY 10964
800-241-1030
www.weleda.com

Personal Insect Repellent
Botanical Solutions, Inc.
PO Box 2070
Southampton, NY 11961
631-287-9700
www.botanicalsolutionsinc.com
Burt's Bees
PO Box 13489
Durham, NC 27709
866-422-8787
www.burtsbees.com
Buzz Away
Quantum
PO Box 2791
Eugene, OR 97402
800-448-1448
www.quantumhealth.com

Pest Control
Beyond Pesticides
701 E Street SE, Suite 200
Washington, DC 20003
202-543-5450
www.beyondpesticides.org

**Northwest Coalition for
Alternatives to Pesticides**
PO Box 1393
Eugene OR 97440-1393
541-344-5044
www.pesticide.org

Pomegranate Juice
POM Wonderful
11444 West Olympic Boulevard
Los Angeles, CA 90064
310-966-5863
www.pomwonderful.com

Rice
Lundberg Family Farms
5370 Church Street
Richvale, CA 95974
530-882-4551
www.lundberg.com

Spices
Frontier Natural Products Co-op
PO Box 299
3021 78th Street
Norway, IA 52318
800-669-3275
www.frontiercoop.com

Sea Vegetables
Gold Mine Natural Foods
7805 Arjons Dr.
San Diego, CA 92126
800-537-9830
www.goldminenaturalfood.com

Seafood and Natural Products
Vital Choice Seafood
605 30th Street
Anacortes, WA 98221
866-482-5887
www.vitalchoice.com

RECOMMENDED READING

Power Healing: Use the New Integrated Medicine to Cure Yourself by Leo Galland, MD (New York: Random House, 1998)

Superimmunity for Kids: What to Feed Your Children to Keep Them Healthy Now—and Prevent Disease in Their Future by Leo Galland, MD (New York: Dell, 1989)

These books by Annie B. Bond offer practical advice on ways to detoxify your home and create a safe, natural environment for you and your family:

Home Enlightenment: Practical, Earth-Friendly Advice for Creating a Nurturing, Healthy, and Toxin-Free Home and Lifestyle. Emmaus, PA: Rodale, 2005.

Better Basics for the Home: Simple Solutions for Less Toxic Living. New York: Three Rivers Press, 1999.

The Green Kitchen Handbook: Practical Advice, References, & Sources for Transforming the Center of Your Home into a Healthy, Livable Place. New York: HarperPerennial, 1997.

Clean and Green: The Complete Guide to Non-Toxic and Environmentally Safe Housekeeping. Woodstock, NY: Ceres Press, 1990.

NOTES

Chapter 1. Your Fat Is Not Your Fault

1. The National Academy of Science News, September 5, 2002. Full report: Dietary Reference Intakes for Energy, Carbohydrate, Fiber, Fat, Fatty Acids, Cholesterol, Protein, and Amino Acids (Macronutrients), A Report of the Panel on Macronutrients, Subcommittees on Upper Reference Levels of Nutrients and Interpretation and Uses of Dietary Reference Intakes, and the Standing Committee on the Scientific Evaluation of Dietary Reference Intakes. National Academy of Sciences, Washington, D.C., 2002. 1408 pages.

2. Horgen, KB, & Brownell, KD. (2002). Confronting the toxic environment: environmental, public health actions in a world crisis. In TA Wadden and AJ Stunkard (Eds.), *Obesity: Theory and Therapy* (2nd edition). New York: Guilford.

Chapter 2. Leptin Resistance: The Reason You Can't Lose Weight

1. Venuta A, Spano C, Laudizi L, Bettelli F, Beverelli A, Turchetto E. Essential fatty acids: the effects of dietary supplementation among children with recurrent respiratory infections. *J Int Med Res*. 1996; 24(4):325–30.

2. Research demonstrating that fat is not inert, but produces hormones known as adipokines: Lafontan M. Fat cells: afferent and efferent messages define new approaches to treat obesity. *Annu Rev Pharmacol Toxicol*. 2005; 45:119–46; Miner JL. The adipocyte as an endocrine cell. *J Anim Sci*. 2004 Mar; 82(3):935–41; Mora S, Pessin JE. An adipocentric view of signaling and intracellular trafficking. *Diabetes Metab Res Rev*. 2002 Sep–Oct; 18(5):345–56; Trayhurn P, Beattie JH. Physiological role of adipose tissue: white adipose tissue as an endocrine and secretory organ. *Proc Nutr Soc*. 2001 Aug; 60(3):329–39.

Research demonstrating that fat regulates itself: Jequier E. Leptin signaling, adiposity, and energy balance. *Ann NY Acad Sci*. 2002 Jun; 967:379–88; Bray GA, York DA. The MONA LISA hypothesis in the time of leptin. *Recent Prog Horm Res*. 1998; 53:95–117.

Research demonstrating that leptin resistance is a key feature of human

obesity: Considine RV, Sinha MK, Heiman ML, et al. Serum immunoreactive-leptin concentrations in normal-weight and obese humans. *N Engl J Med.* 1996; 334:292–95; Caro JF, Sinha MK, Kolaczynski W, Zhang PL, Considine RV. Leptin: the tale of an obesity gene. *Diabetes.* 1996; 45:1455–62; Sinha MK, Caro JF. Clinical aspects of leptin. *Vitam Horm.* 1998; 54:1–30.

3. Zhang Y, Proenca R, Maffei M, Barone M, Leopold L, Friedman JM. Positional cloning of the mouse obese gene and its human homologue. *Nature.* 1994; 372:425–32.

4. Frederich RC, Lollmann B, Hamann A, Napolitano-Rosen A, Kahn BB, Lowell BB, Flier JS. Expression of ob mRNA and its encoded protein in rodents. Impact of nutrition and obesity. *J Clin Invest.* 1995 Sep; 96(3):1658–63.

5. Bajari TM, Nimpf J, Schneider WJ. Role of leptin in reproduction. *Curr Opin Lipidol.* 2004 Jun; 15(3):315–19.

6. Meier U, Gressner AM. Endocrine regulation of energy metabolism: review of pathobiochemical and clinical chemical aspects of leptin, ghrelin, adiponectin, and resistin. *Clin Chem.* 2004 Sep; 50(9):1511–25; Stephens TW, Basinski M, Bristow PK, et al. The role of neuropeptide Y in the antibody action of the *obese* gene product. *Nature.* 1995; 377:530–32; Schwartz MW, Seeley RJ, Woods SC, et al. Leptin increases hypothalamic pro-opiomelanocortin mRNA expression in the rostral arcuate nucleus. *Diabetes.* 1997; 46:2119–23.

7. van Dijk G. The role of leptin in the regulation of energy balance and adiposity. *J Neuroendocrinol.* 2001 Oct; 13(10):913–21; Gullicksen PS, Della-Fera MA, Baile CA. Leptin-induced adipose apoptosis: implications for body weight regulation. *Apoptosis.* 2003 Aug; 8(4):327–35; Wang MY, Lee Y, Unger RH. Novel form of lipolysis induced by leptin. *J Biol Chem.* 1999 Jun 18; 274(25):17541–44.

8. Nedvidkova J, Smitka K, Kopsky V, Hainer V. Adiponectin, an adipocyte-derived protein. *Physiol Res.* 2005; 54(2):133–40.

9. Diez JJ, Iglesias P. The role of the novel adipocyte-derived hormone adiponectin in human disease. *Eur J Endocrinol.* 2003 Mar; 148(3):293–300.

10. Ferre P. Adiponectin: from adipocyte to skeletal muscle. *Ann Endocrinol* (Paris). 2004 Feb; 65(1 Suppl):S36–43; Kamon J, Yamauchi T, Terauchi Y, Kubota N, Kadowaki T. The mechanisms by which PPARgamma and adiponectin regulate glucose and lipid metabolism. *Nippon Yakurigaku Zasshi.* 2003 Oct; 122(4):294–300.

11. Ouchi N, Kihara S, Funahashi T, Matsuzawa Y, Walsh K. Obesity, adiponectin and vascular inflammatory disease. *Curr Opin Lipidol.* 2003 Dec; 14(6):561–66.

12. **Research has also indicated that inflammation inhibits adiponectin synthesis:** Bruun JM, Lihn AS, Verdich C, Pedersen SB, Toubro S, Astrup A, Richelsen B. Regulation of adiponectin by adipose tissue–derived cytokines: in vivo and in vitro investigations in humans. *Am J Physiol Endocrinol Metab.* 2003 Sep; 285(3):E527–33; Fasshauer M, Kralisch S, Klier M, Lossner U, Bluher M, Klein J, Paschke R. Adiponectin gene expression and secretion is inhibited by interleukin-6 in 3T3-L1 adipocytes. *Biochem Biophys Res Commun.* 2003 Feb 21; 301(4):1045–50.

Research demonstrating that leptin increases adiponectin synthesis:

Delporte ML, Ait El Mkadem S, Quisquater M, Brichard SM. Leptin treatment markedly increased plasma adiponectin but barely decreased plasma resistin of ob/ob mice. *Am J Physiol Endocrinol Metab.* 2004 Sep; 287(3):E446–53.

13. Tsuda T, Ueno Y, Aoki H, Koda T, Horio F, Takahashi N, Kawada T, Osawa T. Anthocyanin enhances adipocytokine secretion and adipocyte-specific gene expression in isolated rat adipocytes. *Biochem Biophys Res Commun.* 2004 Mar 26; 316(1):149–57.

14. **Research indicating that inflammation causes chronic degenerative and metabolic disease:** Schmidt MI, Duncan BB. Diabesity: an inflammatory metabolic condition. *Clin Chem Lab Med.* 2003 Sep; 41(9):1120–30; Wisse BE. The inflammatory syndrome: the role of adipose tissue cytokines in metabolic disorders linked to obesity. *J Am Soc Nephrol.* 2004 Nov; 15(11):2792–800; Tracy RP. Emerging relationships of inflammation, cardiovascular disease and chronic diseases of aging. *Int J Obes Relat Metab Disord.* 2003 Dec; 27 Suppl 3:S29–34; Schottenfeld D, Beebe-Dimmer JL. Advances in cancer epidemiology: understanding causal mechanisms and the evidence for implementing interventions. *Annu Rev Public Health.* 2005; 26:37–60.

15. Alexander WS, Hilton DJ. The role of suppressors of cytokine signaling (SOCS) proteins in regulation of the immune response. *Annu Rev Immunol.* 2004; 22:503–29; Elliott J, Johnston JA. SOCS: role in inflammation, allergy and homeostasis. *Trends Immunol.* 2004 Aug; 25(8):434–40; Serhan CN. A search for endogenous mechanisms of anti-inflammation uncovers novel chemical mediators: missing links to resolution. *Histochem Cell Biol.* 2004 Oct; 122(4):305–21.

16. Rakel DP, Rindfleisch A. Inflammation: nutritional, botanical, and mind-body influences. *South Med J.* 2005 Mar; 98(3):303–10.

17. **Research indicating that a high glycemic load is associated with increased C-reactive protein:** Liu S, Manson JE, Buring JE, Stampfer MJ, Willett WC, Ridker PM. Relation between a diet with a high glycemic load and plasma concentrations of high-sensitivity C-reactive protein in middle-aged women. *Am J Clin Nutr.* 2002 Mar; 75(3):492–98.

Research indicating that saturated fat intake is associated with increased C-reactive protein: King DE, Egan BM, Geesey ME. Relation of dietary fat and fiber to elevation of C-reactive protein. *Am J Cardiol.* 2003 Dec 1; 92(11):1335–39.

Research indicating that trans fat consumption is associated with increased C-reactive protein: Mozaffarian D, Pischon T, Hankinson SE, Rifai N, Joshipura K, Willett WC, Rimm EB. Dietary intake of trans fatty acids and systemic inflammation in women. *Am J Clin Nutr.* 2004 Apr; 79(4):606–12; Lopez-Garcia E, Schulze MB, Meigs JB, Manson JE, Rifai N, Stampfer MJ, Willett WC, Hu FB. Consumption of trans fatty acids is related to plasma biomarkers of inflammation and endothelial dysfunction. *J Nutr.* 2005 Mar; 135(3):562–66.

18. Balagopal P, George D, Patton N, Yarandi H, Roberts WL, Bayne E, Gidding S. Lifestyle-only intervention attenuates the inflammatory state associated with obesity: a randomized controlled study in adolescents. *J Pediatr.* 2005 Mar; 146(3):342–48.

19. Seematter G, Binnert C, Martin JL, Tappy L. Relationship between stress, inflammation and metabolism. *Curr Opin Clin Nutr Metab Care.* 2004 Mar; 7(2):169–73; Black PH. The inflammatory response is an integral part of the stress response: Implications for atherosclerosis, insulin resistance, type II diabetes and metabolic syndrome X. *Brain Behav Immun.* 2003 Oct; 17(5):350–64.

20. Girard D. Activation of human polymorphonuclear neutrophils by environmental contaminants. *Rev Environ Health.* 2003 Apr–Jun; 18(2):75–89; Pelletier M, Roberge CJ, Gauthier M, Vandal K, Tessier PA, Girard D. Activation of human neutrophils in vitro and dieldrin-induced neutrophilic inflammation in vivo. *J Leukoc Biol.* 2001 Sep; 70(3):367–73.

21. Das UN. Is obesity an inflammatory condition? *Nutrition.* 2001 Nov–Dec; 17(11–12):953–66.

22. Research on how fat produces inflammatory adipokines: Ferroni P, Basili S, Falco A, Davi G. Inflammation, insulin resistance, and obesity. *Curr Atheroscler Rep.* 2004 Nov; 6(6):424–31; Sonnenberg GE, Krakower GR, Kissebah AH. A novel pathway to the manifestations of metabolic syndrome. *Obes Res.* 2004 Feb; 12(2):180–86.

Research on how inflammation causes insulin resistance: Grimble RF. Inflammatory status and insulin resistance. *Curr Opin Clin Nutr Metab Care.* 2002 Sep; 5(5):551–59; Moller DE. Potential role of TNF-alpha in the pathogenesis of insulin resistance and type 2 diabetes. *Trends Endocrinol Metab.* 2000 Aug; 11(6):212–17.

23. Skurk T, Herder C, Kraft I, Muller-Scholze S, Hauner H, Kolb H. Production and release of macrophage migration inhibitory factor from human adipocytes. *Endocrinology.* 2005 Mar; 146(3):1006–11; Weisberg SP, McCann D, Desai M, Rosenbaum M, Leibel RL, Ferrante AW Jr. Obesity is associated with macrophage accumulation in adipose tissue. *J Clin Invest.* 2003 Dec; 112(12):1796–808.

24. Bjorbaek C, Kahn BB. Leptin signaling in the central nervous system and the periphery. *Recent Prog Horm Res.* 2004; 59:305–31; Wang ZW, Pan WT, Lee Y, Kakuma T, Zhou YT, Unger RH. The role of leptin resistance in the lipid abnormalities of aging. *FASEB J.* 2001 Jan; 15(1):108–14; Bjorbaek C, El-Haschimi K, Frantz JD, Flier JS. The role of SOCS-3 in leptin signaling and leptin resistance. *J Biol Chem.* 1999 Oct 15; 274(42):30059–65; Wang Z, Zhou YT, Kakuma T, Lee Y, Kalra SP, Kalra PS, Pan W, Unger RH. Leptin resistance of adipocytes in obesity: role of suppressors of cytokine signaling. *Biochem Biophys Res Commun.* 2000 Oct 14; 277(1):20–26; Bjorbaek C, Elmquist JK, Frantz JD, Shoelson SE, Flier JS. Identification of SOCS-3 as a potential mediator of central leptin resistance. *Mol Cell.* 1998 Mar; 1(4):619–25.

25. Naslund E, Andersson I, Degerblad M, Kogner P, Kral JG, Rossner S, Hellstrom PM. Associations of leptin, insulin resistance and thyroid function with long-term weight loss in dieting obese men. *J Intern Med.* 2000 Oct; 248(4):299–308.

26. Research on how reduced CRP is associated with higher dietary fiber: Ajani UA, Ford ES, Mokdad AH. Dietary fiber and C-reactive protein: findings from National Health and Nutrition Examination Survey data. *J Nutr.* 2004 May; 134(5):1181–85.

Research on how reduced CRP is associated with higher omega-3 fat intake: Lopez-Garcia E, Schulze MB, Manson JE, Meigs JB, Albert CM, Rifai N, Willett WC, Hu FB. Consumption of (n-3) fatty acids is related to plasma biomarkers of inflammation and endothelial activation in women. *J Nutr.* 2004 Jul; 134(7):1806–11.

Research on the relationship between carotenoids and CRP: Suzuki K, Ito Y, Ochiai J, Kusuhara Y, Hashimoto S, Tokudome S, Kojima M, Wakai K, Toyoshima H, Tamakoshi K, Watanabe Y, Hayakawa N, Maruta M, Watanabe M, Kato K, Ohta Y, Tamakoshi A. JACC Study Group. Relationship between obesity and serum markers of oxidative stress and inflammation in Japanese. *Asian Pac J Cancer Prev.* 2003 Jul–Sep; 4(3):259–66; van Herpen-Broekmans WM, Klopping-Ketelaars IA, Bots ML, Kluft C, Princen H, Hendriks HF, Tijburg LB, van Poppel G, Kardinaal AF. Serum carotenoids and vitamins in relation to markers of endothelial function and inflammation. *Eur J Epidemiol.* 2004; 19(10):915–21; Rowley K, Walker KZ, Cohen J, Jenkins AJ, O'Neal D, Su Q, Best JD, O'Dea K. Inflammation and vascular endothelial activation in an Aboriginal population: relationships to coronary disease risk factors and nutritional markers. *Med J Aust.* 2003 May 19; 178(10):495–500.

27. Sesso HD, Buring JE, Rifai N, Blake GJ, Gaziano JM, Ridker PM. C-reactive protein and the risk of developing hypertension. *JAMA.* 2003 Dec 10; 290(22):2945–51.

28. Blake GJ, Ridker PM. Inflammatory bio-markers and cardiovascular risk prediction. *J Intern Med.* 2002 Oct; 252(4):283–94; Libby P, Ridker PM. Inflammation and atherosclerosis: role of C-reactive protein in risk assessment. *Am J Med.* 2004 Mar 22; 116 Suppl 6A:9S–16S.

29. Penninx BW, Kritchevsky SB, Newman AB, Nicklas BJ, Simonsick EM, Rubin S, Nevitt M, Visser M, Harris T, Pahor M. Inflammatory markers and incident mobility limitation in the elderly. *J Am Geriatr Soc.* 2004 Jul; 52(7):1105–13; Penninx BW, Kritchevsky SB, Yaffe K, Newman AB, Simonsick EM, Rubin S, Ferrucci L, Harris T, Pahor M. Inflammatory markers and depressed mood in older persons: results from the Health, Aging and Body Composition study. *Biol Psychiatry.* 2003 Sep 1; 54(5):566–72.

30. de Maat MP, Kluft C. Determinants of C-reactive protein concentration in blood. *Ital Heart J.* 2001 Mar; 2(3):189–95; Kazumi T, Kawaguchi A, Hirano T, Yoshino G. C-reactive protein in young, apparently healthy men: associations with serum leptin, QTc interval, and high-density lipoprotein-cholesterol. *Metabolism.* 2003 Sep; 52(9):1113–16.

31. Esposito K, Marfella R, Ciotola M, Di Palo C, Giugliano F, Giugliano G, D'Armiento M, D'Andrea F, Giugliano D. Effect of a Mediterranean-style diet on endothelial dysfunction and markers of vascular inflammation in the metabolic syndrome: a randomized trial. *JAMA.* 2004 Sep 22; 292(12):1440–46.

32. Shamsuzzaman AMS, Winnicki M, Wolk R, et al. Independent association between plasma leptin and c-reactive protein in healthy humans. *Circulation.* 2004; 109:2181-2185.

33. Kazumi T, Kawaguchi A, Hirano T, Yoshino G. C-reactive protein in

young, apparently healthy men: associations with serum leptin, QTc interval, and high-density lipoprotein-cholesterol. *Metabolism*. 2003; 52:1113-6.

34. Ble A, Windham BG, Bandinelli S, et al. Relation of plasma leptin to C-reactive protein in older adults (from the Invecchiare nel Chianti study). *Am J Cardiol*. 2005; 96: 991-5.

35. Bulló M, García-Lorda P, Megias I, Salas-Salvadó J. Systemic inflammation, adipose tissue tumor necrosis factor, and leptin expression. *Obes Res*. 2003; 11:525-31.

36. Chen K, Li F, Li J, Cai H, et al. Induction of leptin resistance through direct interaction of C-reactive protein with leptin. *Nat Med*. 2006; 12: 425-32.

37. Steinberg GR, McAinch AJ, Chen MB, et al. The suppressor of cytokine signaling 3 inhibits leptin activation of AMP-kinase in cultured skeletal muscle of obese humans. *J Clin Endocrinol Metab*. 2006; 91:3592-7.

38. Howard JK, Flier JS. Attentuation of leptin and insulin signaling by SOCS proteins. *Trends Endocrinol Metab*. 2006; 17: 365-71.

Chapter 3. The Real Truth About Fats

1. Lau CS, Morley KD, Belch JJ. Effects of fish oil supplementation on non-steroidal anti-inflammatory drug requirement in patients with mild rheumatoid arthritis—a double-blind placebo controlled study. *Br J Rheumatol*. 1993 Nov; 32(11):982–89; Kremer JN. n-3 fatty acid supplements in rheumatoid arthritis. *Am J Clin Nutr*. 2000 Jan; 71(1 Suppl):349S–51S; Cleland LG, James MJ, Proudman SM. Omega-6/omega-3 fatty acids and arthritis. *World Rev Nutr Diet*. 2003; 92:152–68; Adam O, Beringer C, Kless T, Lemmen C, Adam A, Wiseman M, Adam P, Klimmek R, Forth W. Anti-inflammatory effects of a low arachidonic acid diet and fish oil in patients with rheumatoid arthritis. *Rheumatol Int*. 2003 Jan; 23(1):27–36.

2. Baer DJ, Judd JT, Clevidence BA, Tracy RP. Dietary fatty acids affect plasma markers of inflammation in healthy men fed controlled diets: a randomized crossover study. *Am J Clin Nutr*. 2004 Jun; 79(6):969–73; Pirro M, Schillaci G, Savarese G, Gemelli F, Mannarino MR, Siepi D, Bagaglia F, Mannarino E. Attenuation of inflammation with short-term dietary intervention is associated with a reduction of arterial stiffness in subjects with hypercholesterolaemia. *Eur J Cardiovasc Prev Rehabil*. 2004 Dec; 11(6):497–502; King DE, Egan BM, Geesey ME. Relation of dietary fat and fiber to elevation of C-reactive protein. *Am J Cardiol*. 2003 Dec 1; 92(11):1335–39.

Research also indicates that saturated fat can cause insulin resistance: Vessby B, Unsitupa M, Hermansen K, Riccardi G, Rivellese AA, Tapsell LC, Nalsen C, Berglund L, Louheranta A, Rasmussen BM, Calvert GD, Maffetone A, Pedersen E, Gustafsson IB, Storlien LH. KANWU Study. Substituting dietary saturated for monounsaturated fat impairs insulin sensitivity in healthy men and women: the KANWU Study. *Diabetologia*. 2001 Mar; 44(3):312–19.

3. Lopez-Garcia E, Schulze MB, Manson JE, Meigs JB, Albert CM, Rifai N, Willett WC, Hu FB. Consumption of (n-3) fatty acids is related to plasma bio-

markers of inflammation and endothelial activation in women. *J Nutr.* 2004 Jul; 134(7):1806–11; Mori TA, Beilin LJ. Omega-3 fatty acids and inflammation. *Curr Atheroscler Rep.* 2004 Nov; 6(6):461–67.

4. de Lorgeril M, Salen P. Alpha-linolenic acid and coronary heart disease. *Nutr Metab Cardiovasc Dis.* 2004 Jun; 14(3):162–69.

5. Rakel DP, Rindfleisch A. Inflammation: nutritional, botanical, and mind-body influences. *South Med J.* 2005 Mar; 98(3):303–10; Simopoulos AP. The importance of the ratio of omega-6/omega-3 essential fatty acids. *Biomed Pharmacother.* 2002 Oct; 56(8):365–79; Simopoulos AP. Human requirement for N-3 polyunsaturated fatty acids. *Poult Sci.* 2000 Jul; 79(7):961–70; Simopoulos AP. Importance of the ratio of omega-6/omega-3 essential fatty acids: evolutionary aspects. *World Rev Nutr Diet.* 2003; 92:1–22.

6. Oh K, Hu FB, Manson JE, Stampfer MJ, Willett WC. Dietary fat intake and risk of coronary heart disease in women: 20 years of follow-up of the nurses' health study. *Am J Epidemiol.* 2005 Apr 1; 161(7):672–79; Hu FB, Stampfer MJ, Manson JE, Rimm E, Colditz GA, Rosner BA, Hennekens CH, Willett WC. Dietary fat intake and the risk of coronary heart disease in women. *N Engl J Med.* 1997 Nov 20; 337(21):1491–99; de Roos NM, Schouten EG, Scheek LM, van Tol A, Katan MB. Replacement of dietary saturated fat with trans fat reduces serum paraoxonase activity in healthy men and women. *Metabolism.* 2002 Dec; 51(12):1534–37.

7. Lopez-Garcia E, Schulze MB, Meigs JB, Manson JE, Rifai N, Stampfer MJ, Willett WC, Hu FB. Consumption of trans fatty acids is related to plasma bio-markers of inflammation and endothelial dysfunction. *J Nutr.* 2005 Mar; 135(3):562–66; Mozaffarian D, Rimm EB, King IB, Lawler RL, McDonald GB, Levy WC. Trans fatty acids and systemic inflammation in heart failure. *Am J Clin Nutr.* 2004 Dec; 80(6):1521–25; Baer DJ, Judd JT, Clevidence BA, Tracy RP. Dietary fatty acids affect plasma markers of inflammation in healthy men fed controlled diets: a randomized crossover study. *Am J Clin Nutr.* 2004 Jun; 79(6):969–73.

8. Koh-Banerjee P, Chu NF, Spiegelman D, Rosner B, Colditz G, Willett W, Rimm E. Prospective study of the association of changes in dietary intake, physical activity, alcohol consumption, and smoking with 9-year gain in waist circumference among 16 587 US men. *Am J Clin Nutr.* 2003 Oct; 78(4):719–27.

9. Eaton SB, Konner M. Paleolithic nutrition. A consideration of its nature and current implications. *N Engl J Med.* 1985 Jan 31; 312(5):283–89.

Chapter 4. The Real Truth About Carbs

1. Singh RB, Niaz MA, Ghosh S. Effect on central obesity and associated disturbances of low-energy, fruit- and vegetable-enriched prudent diet in north Indians. *Postgrad Med J.* 1994 Dec; 70(830):895–900.

2. Serra I, Yamamoto M, Calvo A, Cavada G, Baez S, Endoh K, Watanabe H, Tajima K. Association of chili pepper consumption, low socioeconomic status and longstanding gallstones with gallbladder cancer in a Chilean population. *Int J*

Cancer. 2002 Dec 1; 102(4):407–11; Pandey M, Shukla VK. Diet and gallbladder cancer: a case-control study. *Eur J Cancer Prev.* 2002 Aug; 11(4):365–68; Mathew A, Gangadharan P, Varghese C, Nair MK. Diet and stomach cancer: a case-control study in South India. *Eur J Cancer Prev.* 2000 Apr; 9(2):89–97; Lopez-Carrillo L, Lopez-Cervantes M, Robles-Diaz G, Ramirez-Espitia A, Mohar-Betancourt A, Meneses-Garcia A, Lopez-Vidal Y, Blair A. Capsaicin consumption, Helicobacter pylori positivity and gastric cancer in Mexico. *Int J Cancer.* 2003 Aug 20; 106(2):277–82; Surh YJ, Lee SS. Capsaicin in hot chili pepper: carcinogen, co-carcinogen or anticarcinogen? *Food Chem Toxicol.* 1996 Mar; 34(3):313–16.

3. Reilly CA, Taylor JL, Lanza DL, Carr BA, Crouch DJ, Yost GS. Capsaicinoids cause inflammation and epithelial cell death through activation of vanilloid receptors. *Toxicol Sci.* 2003 May; 73(1):170–81. Geppetti P, Trevisani M. Activation and sensitisation of the vanilloid receptor: role in gastrointestinal inflammation and function. *Br J Pharmacol.* 2004 Apr; 141(8):1313–20.

4. Lambert JD, Hong J, Kim DH, Mishin VM, Yang CS. Piperine enhances the bioavailability of the tea polyphenol (-)-epigallocatechin-3-gallate in mice. *J Nutr.* 2004 Aug; 134(8):1948–52; Shoba G, Joy D, Joseph T, Majeed M, Rajendran R, Srinivas PS. Influence of piperine on the pharmacokinetics of curcumin in animals and human volunteers. *Planta Med.* 1998 May; 64(4):353–56.

5. Lampe JW. Spicing up a vegetarian diet: chemopreventive effects of phytochemicals. *Am J Clin Nutr.* 2003 Sep; 78(3 Suppl):579S–583S; Heber D. Vegetables, fruits and phytoestrogens in the prevention of diseases. *J Postgrad Med.* 2004 Apr-Jun; 50(2):145–49; Youdim KA, McDonald J, Kalt W, Joseph JA. Potential role of dietary flavonoids in reducing microvascular endothelium vulnerability to oxidative and inflammatory insults. *J Nutr Biochem.* 2002 May; 13(5):282–88; Cos P, De Bruyne T, Hermans N, Apers S, Berghe DV, Vlietinck AJ. Proanthocyanidins in health care: current and new trends. *Curr Med Chem.* 2004 May; 11(10):1345–59; Aggarwal BB, Shishodia S. Suppression of the nuclear factor-κB activation pathway by spice-derived phytochemicals: reasoning for seasoning. *Ann NY Acad Sci.* 2004 Dec; 1030:434–41.

Research on garlic: Hodge G, Hodge S, Han P. Allium sativum (garlic) suppresses leukocyte inflammatory cytokine production in vitro: potential therapeutic use in the treatment of inflammatory bowel disease. *Cytometry.* 2002 Aug 1; 48(4):209–15; Hofbauer R, Frass M, Gmeiner B, Kaye AD, Frost EA. Effects of garlic extract (Allium sativum) on neutrophil migration at the cellular level. *Heart Dis.* 2001 Jan-Feb; 3(1):14–17.

Research on ginger: Ozaki Y, Kawahara N, Harada M. Anti-inflammatory effect of *Zingiber cassumunar Roxb.* and its active principles. *Chem Pharm Bull* (Tokyo). 1991; 39:2353–56.

Research on turmeric: Plummer SM, Holloway KA, Manson MM, et al. Inhibition of cyclo-oxygenase 2 expression in colon cells by the chemopreventive agent curcumin involves inhibition of NF-κB activation via the NIK/IKK signalling complex. *Oncogene.* 1999; 18:6013–20; Jobin C, Bradham CA, Russo MP,

Juma B, Narula AS, Brenner DA, Sartor RB. Curcumin blocks cytokine-mediated NF-kappa B activation and proinflammatory gene expression by inhibiting inhibitory factor I-kappa B kinase activity. *J Immunol.* 1999 Sep 15; 163(6):3474–83.

Research on onions: Dorsch W, Schneider E, Bayer T, Breu W, Wagner H. Anti-inflammatory effects of onions: inhibition of chemotaxis of human polymorphonuclear leukocytes by thiosulfinates and cepaenes. *Int Arch Allergy Appl Immunol.* 1990; 92(1):39–42.

Research on parsley: Nielsen SE, Young JF, Daneshvar B, Lauridsen ST, Knuthsen P, Sandstrom B, Dragsted LO. Effect of parsley (Petroselinum crispum) intake on urinary apigenin excretion, blood antioxidant enzymes and biomarkers for oxidative stress in human subjects. *Br J Nutr.* 1999 Jun; 81(6):447–55.

Research on basil: Singh S. Mechanism of action of anti-inflammatory effect of fixed oil of Ocimum basilicum Linn. *Indian J Exp Biol.* 1999 Mar; 37(3):248–52.

Research on cherries: Tall JM, Seeram NP, Zhao C, Nair MG, Meyer RA, Raja SN. Tart cherry anthocyanins suppress inflammation-induced pain behavior in rat. *Behav Brain Res.* 2004 Aug 12; 153(1):181–88; Blando F, Gerardi C, Nicoletti I. Sour cherry (Prunus cerasus L) anthocyanins as ingredients for functional foods. *J Biomed Biotechnol.*; 2004(5):253–258; Wang HB, Nair MG, Strasburg GM, Chang YC, Booren AM, Gray JI, DeWitt DL. Antioxidant and anti-inflammatory activities of anthocyanins and their aglycon, cyanidin, from tart cherries. *J Nat Prod.* 1999; 62:294–296

Research on pomegranates: Schubert SY, Neeman I, Resnick N. A novel mechanism for the inhibition of NF-kappa B activation in vascular endothelial cells by natural antioxidants. *FASEB J.* 2002 Dec; 16(14):1931–33; Afaq F, Malik A, Syed D, Maes D, Matsui MS, Mukhtar H. Pomegranate fruit extract modulates UV-B-mediated phosphorylation of mitogen-activated protein kinases and activation of nuclear factor kappa B in normal human epidermal keratinocytes paragraph sign. *Photochem Photobiol.* 2005 Jan-Feb; 81(1):38–45.

Research on green tea: Hofbauer R, Frass M, Gmeiner B, Handler S, Speiser W, Kapiotis S. The green tea extract epigallocatechin gallate is able to reduce neutrophil transmigration through monolayers of endothelial cells. *Wien Klin Wochenschr.* 1999 Apr 9; 111(7):278–82.

Research on black tea: Lin YL, Tsai SH, Lin-Shiau SY, Ho CT, Lin JK. Theaflavin-3,3′-digallate from black tea blocks the nitric oxide synthase by down-regulating the activation of NF-kappa B in macrophages. *Eur J Pharmacol.* 1999 Feb 19; 367(2–3):379–88.

6. Cavadini C, Siega-Riz AM, Popkin BM. US adolescent food intake trends from 1965 to 1996. *Arch Dis Child.* 2000 Jul; 83(1):18–24. (Potatoes accounted for 50 percent of alleged vegetable consumption in 1996.)

7. Liu S, Manson JE, Buring JE, Stampfer MJ, Willett WC, Ridker PM. Relation between a diet with a high glycemic load and plasma concentrations of high-sensitivity C-reactive protein in middle-aged women. *Am J Clin Nutr.* 2002 Mar; 75(3):492–98.

8. Jensen MK, Koh-Banerjee P, Hu FB, Franz M, Sampson L, Gronbaek M, Rimm EB. Intakes of whole grains, bran, and germ and the risk of coronary heart

disease in men. *Am J Clin Nutr.* 2004 Dec; 80(6):1492–99; Lupton JR, Turner ND. Dietary fiber and coronary disease: does the evidence support an association? *Curr Atheroscler. Rep* 2003 Nov; 5(6):500–5; Gariballa SE. Nutritional factors in stroke. *Br J Nutr.* 2000 Jul; 84(1):5–17; Martinez ME. Primary prevention of colorectal cancer: lifestyle, nutrition, exercise. *Recent Results Cancer Res.* 2005; 166:177–211; Tseng M, Everhart JE, Sandler RS. Dietary intake and gallbladder disease: a review. *Public Health Nutr.* 1999 Jun; 2(2):161–72.

9. Ajani UA, Ford ES, Mokdad AH. Dietary fiber and C-reactive protein: findings from national health and nutrition examination survey data. *J Nutr.* 2004 May; 134(5):1181–85.

10. Suzuki K, Ito Y, Ochiai J, Kusuhara Y, Hashimoto S, Tokudome S, Kojima M, Wakai K, Toyoshima H, Tamakoshi K, Watanabe Y, Hayakawa N, Maruta M, Watanabe M, Kato K, Ohta Y, Tamakoshi A. JACC study group. Relationship between obesity and serum markers of oxidative stress and inflammation in Japanese. *Asian Pac J Cancer Prev.* 2003 Jul-Sep; 4(3):259–66; van Herpen-Broekmans WM, Klopping-Ketelaars IA, Bots ML, Kluft C, Princen H, Hendriks HF, Tijburg LB, van Poppel G, Kardinaal AF. Serum carotenoids and vitamins in relation to markers of endothelial function and inflammation. *Eur J Epidemiol.* 2004; 19(10):915–21; Rowley K, Walker KZ, Cohen J, Jenkins AJ, O'Neal D, Su Q, Best JD, O'Dea K. Inflammation and vascular endothelial activation in an Aboriginal population: relationships to coronary disease risk factors and nutritional markers. *Med J Aust.* 2003 May 19; 178(10):495–500; Kim HP, Son KH, Chang HW, Kang SS. Anti-inflammatory plant flavonoids and cellular action mechanisms. *J Pharmacol Sci.* 2004 Nov; 96(3):229–45; Horvathova K, Vachalkova A, Novotny L. Flavonoids as chemoprotective agents in civilization diseases. *Neoplasma.* 2001; 48(6):435–41; Manthey JA. Biological properties of flavonoids pertaining to inflammation. *Microcirculation.* 2000; 7(6 Pt 2):S29–3; Middleton E Jr, Kandaswami C, Theoharides TC. The effects of plant flavonoids on mammalian cells: implications for inflammation, heart disease, and cancer. *Pharmacol Rev.* 2000 Dec; 52(4):673–751; Middleton E Jr. Effect of plant flavonoids on immune and inflammatory cell function. *Adv Exp Med Biol.* 1998; 439:175–82.

11. Esmaillzadeh A, Tahbaz F, Gaieni I, Alavi-Majd H, Azadbakht L. Concentrated pomegranate juice improves lipid profiles in diabetic patients with hyperlipidemia. *J Med Food.* 2004 Fall; 7(3):305–8; Aviram M, Rosenblat M, Gaitini D, Nitecki S, Hoffman A, Dornfeld L, Volkova N, Presser D, Attias J, Liker H, Hayek T. Pomegranate juice consumption for 3 years by patients with carotid artery stenosis reduces common carotid intima-media thickness and blood pressure, and protects against LDL oxidation. *Clin Nutr.* 2004 Jun; 23(3):423–33.

12. Joseph JA, Shukitt-Hale B, Casadesus G. Reversing the deleterious effects of aging on neuronal communication and behavior: beneficial properties of fruit polyphenolic compounds. *Am J Clin Nutr.* 2005 Jan; 81(1 Suppl): 313S–16S.

13. Blau LW. Cherry diet control for gout and arthritis. *Tex Rep Biol Med.* 1950; 8(3):309–11.

14. Ambrosone CB, McCann SE, Freudenheim JL, Marshall JR, Zhang Y,

Shields PG. Breast cancer risk in premenopausal women is inversely associated with consumption of broccoli, a source of isothiocyanates, but is not modified by GST genotype. *J Nutr.* 2004 May; 134(5):1134–38.

15. Hsing AW, Chokkalingam AP, Gao YT, Madigan MP, Deng J, Gridley G, Fraumeni JF Jr. Allium vegetables and risk of prostate cancer: a population-based study. *J Natl Cancer Inst.* 2002 Nov 6; 94(21):1648–51.

16. Mustafa T, Srivastava KC. Ginger (Zingiber officinale) in migraine headache. *J Ethnopharmacol.* 1990 Jul; 29(3):267–73; Fischer-Rasmussen W, Kjaer SK, Dahl C, Asping U. Ginger treatment of hyperemesis gravidarum. *Eur J Obstet Gynecol Reprod Biol.* 1991 Jan 4; 38(1):19–24; Altman RD, Marcussen KC. Effects of a ginger extract on knee pain in patients with osteoarthritis. *Arthritis Rheum.* 2001 Nov; 44(11):2531–38; Kiuchi F, Iwakami S, Shibuya M, Hanaoka F, Sankawa U. Inhibition of prostaglandin and leukotriene biosynthesis by gingerols and diarylheptanoids. *Chem Pharm Bull* (Tokyo). 1992 Feb; 40(2):387–91.

17. Aggarwal BB, Kumar A, Bharti AC. Anticancer potential of curcumin: preclinical and clinical studies. *Anticancer Res.* 2003 Jan-Feb; 23(1A):363–98; Dinkova-Kostova AT. Protection against cancer by plant phenylpropenoids: induction of mammalian anticarcinogenic enzymes. *Mini Rev Med Chem.* 2002 Dec; 2(6):595–610.

18. Research has also demonstrated that cinnamon appears to increase insulin sensitivity: Anderson RA, Broadhurst CL, Polansky MM, Schmidt WF, Khan A, Flanagan VP, Schoene NW, Graves DJ. Isolation and characterization of polyphenol type-A polymers from cinnamon with insulin-like biological activity. *J Agric Food Chem.* 2004; 52(1):65–70.

19. Staprans I, Pan XM, Rapp JH, Feingold KR. Oxidized cholesterol in the diet is a source of oxidized lipoproteins in human serum. *J Lipid Res.* 2003 Apr; 44(4):705–15; Ursini F, Sevanian A. Postprandial oxidative stress. *Biol Chem* 2002 Mar-Apr; 383(3–4):599–605; Weisburger JH. Mechanisms of action of antioxidants as exemplified in vegetables, tomatoes and tea. *Food Chem Toxicol.* 1999 Sep-Oct; 37(9–10):943–48.

Chapter 5. What's Wrong with Other Diets?

1. Steward LH, Bethea M, Andrews S. *Sugar Busters! Cut Sugar to Trim Fat.* Ballantine, New York, 1998. 288 pages.

2. Lin L, Martin R, Schaffhauser AO, York DA. Acute changes in the response to peripheral leptin with alteration in the diet composition. *Am J Physiol Regul Integr Comp Physiol.* 2001 Feb; 280(2):R504–9.

3. Foster GD, Wyatt HR, Hill JO, McGuckin BG, Brill C, Mohammed BS, Szapary PO, Rader DJ, Edman JS, Klein S. A randomized trial of a low-carbohydrate diet for obesity. *N Engl J Med.* 2003 May 22; 348(21):2082–90; Dansinger ML, Gleason JA, Griffith JL, Selker HP, Schaefer EJ. Comparison of the Atkins, Ornish, Weight Watchers, and Zone diets for weight loss and heart disease risk reduction: a randomized trial. *JAMA.* 2005 Jan 5; 293(1):43–53.

4. Woods SC, Benoit SC, Clegg DJ, Seeley RJ. Clinical endocrinology and

metabolism. Regulation of energy homeostasis by peripheral signals. *Best Pract Res Clin Endocrinol Metab.* 2004 Dec; 18(4):497–515; Laville M, Cornu C, Normand S, Mithieux G, Beylot M, Riou JP. Decreased glucose-induced thermogenesis at the onset of obesity. *Am J Clin Nutr.* 1993 Jun; 57(6):851–56; Golay A. Blunted glucose-induced thermogenesis: a factor contributing to relapse of obesity. *Int J Obes Relat Metab Disord.* 1993 Feb; 17 Suppl 1:S23–27.

5. Carvalheira JB, Siloto RM, Ignacchitti I, Brenelli SL, Carvalho CR, Leite A, Velloso LA, Gontijo JA, Saad MJ. Insulin modulates leptin-induced STAT3 activation in rat hypothalamus. *FEBS Lett.* 2001 Jul 6; 500(3):119–24.

6. Manco M, Calvani M, Mingrone G. Effects of dietary fatty acids on insulin sensitivity and secretion. *Diabetes Obes Metab.* 2004; 6(6):402–13.

7. Yang MU, Van Itallie TB. Composition of weight lost during short-term weight reduction. Metabolic responses of obese subjects to starvation and low-calorie ketogenic and nonketogenic diets. *J Clin Invest.* 1976 Sep; 58(3):722–30; Bilsborough SA, Crowe TC. Low-carbohydrate diets: what are the potential short- and long-term health implications? *Asia Pac J Clin Nutr.* 2003; 12(4):396–404.

8. Reddy ST, Wang CY, Sakhaee K, Brinkley L, Pak CY. Effect of low-carbohydrate high-protein diets on acid-base balance, stone-forming propensity, and calcium metabolism. *Am J Kidney Dis.* 2002 Aug; 40(2):265–74.

9. Butki BD, Baumstark J, Driver S. Effects of a carbohydrate-restricted diet on affective responses to acute exercise among physically active participants. *Percept Mot Skills.* 2003 Apr; 96(2):607–15.

10. Segal-Isaacson CJ, Johnson S, Tomuta V, Cowell B, Stein DT. A randomized trial comparing low-fat and low-carbohydrate diets matched for energy and protein. *Obes Res.* 2004 Nov; 12 Suppl 2:130S–40S.

11. Agatston, A. *The South Beach Diet: The Foolproof, Doctor-Designed Plan for Fast and Healthy Weight Loss.* Rodale, Emmaus, Pa., 2003. 320 pages.

Chapter 6. The Fat Resistance Eating Plan

1. Sheard NF. Fish consumption and risk of sudden cardiac death. Nutr Rev. 1998; 56(6):177–79; Morris MC, Evans DA, Bienias JL, Tangney CC, Bennett DA, Wilson RS, Aggarwal N, Schneider J. Consumption of fish and n-3 fatty acids and risk of incident Alzheimer disease. *Arch Neurol.* 2003; 60(7):940–46.

2. Ajani UA, Ford ES, Mokdad AH, Dietary fiber and C-reactive protein: findings from National Health and Nutrition Examination Survey data. *J Nutr.* 2004; 134(5):1181–85.

3. Bazzano LA, He J, Ogden LG, Loria CM, Whelton PK; National Health and Nutrition Examination Survey I Epidemiologic Follow-up Study. Dietary fiber intake and reduced risk of coronary heart disease in US men and women: the National Health and Nutrition Examination Survey I Epidemiologic Follow-up Study. *Arch Intern Med.* 2003 Sep 8; 163(16):1897–904; Liu S, Manson JE, Stampfer MJ, Rexrode KM, Hu FB, Rimm EB, Willett WC. Whole grain consumption and risk of ischemic stroke in women: a prospective study. *JAMA.* 2000;

284(12):1534–40; Oh K, Hu FB, Cho E, Rexrode KM, Stampfer MJ, Manson JE, Liu S, Willett WC. Carbohydrate intake, glycemic index, glycemic load, and dietary fiber in relation to risk of stroke in women. *Am J Epidemiol.* 2005; 161(2):161–69; Williams GM, Williams CL, Weisburg JH. Diet and cancer prevention: the fiber first diet. *Toxicol Sci.* 1999; 52(2 Suppl):72–86; Campos FG, Logullo Waitzberg AG, Kiss DR, Waitzberg DL, Habr-Gama A, Gama-Rodrigues J. Diet and colorectal cancer: current evidence for etiology and prevention. *Nutr Hosp.* 2005; 20(1):18–25.

4. Yao LH, Jiang YM, Shi J, Tomas-Barberan FA, Datta N, Singanusong R, Chen SS. Flavonoids in food and their health benefits. *Plant Foods Hum Nutr.* 2004 Summer; 59(3):113–22; Hertog MG, Feskens EJ, Hollman PC, Katan MB, Kromhout D. Dietary antioxidant flavonoids and risk of coronary heart disease: the Zutphen Elderly Study. *Lancet.* 1993; 342(8878):1007–11; Keli SO, Hertog MG, Feskens EJ, Kromhout D. Dietary flavonoids, antioxidant vitamins, and incidence of stroke: the Zutphen study. *Arch Intern Med.* 1996; 156(6):637–42.

5. Brown MJ, Ferruzzi MG, Nguyen ML. Carotenoid bioavailability is higher from salads ingested with full-fat than with fat-reduced dressings as measured with electrochemical detection. *Am J Clin Nutr.* 2004 Aug; 60:396–403.

6. Snowdon DA. Animal product consumption and mortality because of all causes combined, coronary heart disease, stroke, diabetes, and cancer in Seventh-Day Adventists. *Am J Clin Nutr.* 1988 Sep; 48(3 Suppl):739–48.

7. Brown MJ, Ferruzzi MG, Nguyen ML. Carotenoid bioavailability is higher from salads ingested with full-fat than with fat-reduced dressings as measured with electrochemical detection. *Am J Clin Nutr.* 2004 Aug; 60:396–403.

8. Lappe JM, Travers-Gustafson D, Davies KM, Recker RR, Heaney RP. Vitamin D and calcium supplementation reduces cancer risk: results of a randomized trial. *Am J Clin Nutr.* 2007 Jun; 85(6):1586–91

9. Rodriguez-Stanley S, Ahmed T, Zubaidi S, Riley S, Akbarali HI, Mellow MH, Miner PB. Calcium carbonate antacids alter esophageal motility in heartburn sufferers. *Dig Dis Sci.* 2004 Nov-Dec; 49(11-12):1862-7.

10. Akaogi J, Barker T, Kuroda Y, Nacionales DC, Yamasaki Y, Stevens BR, Reeves WH, Satoh M. Role of non-protein amino acid L-canavanine in autoimmunity. *Autoimmun Rev.* 2006 Jul; 5(6):429-35.

11. Watanabe K, Reddy BS, Weisburger JH, Kritchevsky D. Effect of dietary alfalfa, pectin, and wheat bran on azoxymethane- or methylnitrosourea-induced colon carcinogenesis in F344 rats. *J Natl Cancer Inst.* 1979 Jul; 63(1):141-5.

12. Maeda H, Hosokawa M, Sashima T, Miyashita K. Dietary combination of fucoxanthin and fish oil attenuates the weight gain of white adipose tissue and decreases blood glucose in obese/diabetic KK-A(y)mice. *J Agric Food Chem.* 2007 Aug 23.

13. Yoshiko S, Hoyoku N. Fucoxanthin, a natural carotenoid, induces G1 arrest and GADD45 gene expression in human cancer cells. *In Vivo.* 2007 Mar-Apr; 21(2):305-9.

14. Blackburn GL. Low-calorie protein versus mixed diet. *N Engl J Med.* 1980; 303(3):158.

15. Halton TL, Hu FB. The effects of high protein diets on thermogenesis, satiety and weight loss: a critical review. *J Am Coll Nutr.* 2004; 23(5):373–85.

Chapter 7. The Joy of Movement:
How Exercise Can Help You Overcome Leptin Resistance

1. Wing RR, Hill JO. Successful weight loss maintenance. *Annu Rev Nutr.* 2001; 21:323–41; Klem ML, Wing RR, McGuire MT, Seagle HM, Hill JO. A descriptive study of individuals successful at long-term maintenance of substantial weight loss. *Am J Clin Nutr.* 1997 Aug; 66(2):239–46; McGuire MT, Wing RR, Klem ML, Seagle HM, Hill JO. Long-term maintenance of weight loss: do people who lose weight through various weight loss methods use different behaviors to maintain their weight? *Int J Obes Relat Metab Disord.* 1998 Jun; 22(6):572–77.

2. DiLorenzo TM, Bargman EP, Stucky-Ropp R, Brassington GS, Frensch PA, LaFontaine T. Long-term effects of aerobic exercise on psychological outcomes. *Prev Med.* 1999 Jan; 28(1):75–85; Nieman DC. Current perspective on exercise immunology. *Curr Sports Med Rep.* 2003 Oct; 2(5):239–42.

3. Colbert LH, Visser M, Simonsick EM, Tracy RP, Newman AB, Kritchevsky SB, Pahor M, Taaffe DR, Brach J, Rubin S, Harris TB. Physical activity, exercise, and inflammatory markers in older adults: findings from the Health, Aging and Body Composition Study. *J Am Geriatr Soc.* 2004 Jul; 52(7):1098–104; Wegge JK, Roberts CK, Ngo TH, Barnard RJ. Effect of diet and exercise intervention on inflammatory and adhesion molecules in postmenopausal women on hormone replacement therapy and at risk for coronary artery disease. *Metabolism.* 2004 Mar; 53(3):377–81; King DE, Carek P, Mainous AG 3rd, Pearson WS. Inflammatory markers and exercise: differences related to exercise type. *Med Sci Sports Exerc.* 2003 Apr; 35(4):575–81.

4. Chu NF, Stampfer MJ, Spiegelman D, Rifai N, Hotamisligil GS, Rimm EB. Dietary and lifestyle factors in relation to plasma leptin concentrations among normal weight and overweight men. *Int J Obes Relat Metab Disord.* 2001 Jan; 25(1):106–14.

5. World Health Organization. Diet, nutrition and the prevention of chronic diseases. *World Health Organ Tech Rep Ser.* 2003; 916:i–viii, 1–149.

6. Eaton SB, Eaton SB. An evolutionary perspective on human physical activity: implications for health. *Comp Biochem Physiol A Mol Integr Physiol.* 2003 Sep; 136(1):153–59.

7. Tudor-Locke C, Ainsworth BE, Whitt MC, Thompson RW, Addy CL, Jones DA. The relationship between pedometer-determined ambulatory activity and body composition variables. *Int J Obes Relat Metab Disord.* 2001 Nov; 25(11):1571–78.

8. Thompson DL, Rakow J, Perdue SM. Relationship between accumulated walking and body composition in middle-aged women. *Med Sci Sports Exerc.* 2004 May; 36(5):911–14.

9. Suzuki K, Nakaji S, Yamada M, Totsuka M, Sato K, Sugawara K. Systemic inflammatory response to exhaustive exercise. Cytokine kinetics. *Exerc Immunol*

Rev. 2002; 8:6–48; Meyer T, Gabriel HH, Ratz M, Muller HJ, Kindermann W. Anaerobic exercise induces moderate acute phase response. *Med Sci Sports Exerc.* 2001 Apr; 33(4):549–55.

Chapter 8. Relaxing into a Healthy Weight

1. Kripke DF, Garfinkel L, Wingard DL, Klauber MR, Marler MR. Mortality associated with sleep duration and insomnia. *Arch Gen Psychiatry.* 2002; 59:131–36; Taheri S, Lin L, Austin D, Young T, Mignot E. Short sleep duration is associated with reduced leptin, elevated ghrelin, and increased body mass index. *PLoS Med.* 2004 Dec; 1(3):e62.

2. Yudkin JS, Kumari M, Humphries SE, Mohamed-Ali V. Inflammation, obesity, stress and coronary heart disease: is interleukin-6 the link? *Atherosclerosis.* 2000 Feb; 148(2):209–14.

3. Rosmond R. Stress-induced disturbances of the HPA axis: a pathway to Type 2 diabetes? *Med Sci Monit.* 2003 Feb; 9(2):RA35–39; Bjorntorp P. Neuroendocrine perturbations as a cause of insulin resistance. *Diabetes Metab Res Rev.* 1999 Nov–Dec; 15(6):427–41.

4. Fasshauer M, Klein J, Neumann S, Eszlinger M, Paschke R. Constitutive activation of STAT-3 and downregulation of SOCS-3 expression induced by adrenalectomy. *Am J Physiol Regul Integr Comp Physiol.* 2001 Dec; 281(6):R2048–58.

5. Fasshauer M, Klein J, Neumann S, Eszlinger M, Paschke R. Hormonal regulation of adiponectin gene expression in 3T3-L1 adipocytes. *Biochem Biophys Res Commun.* 2002 Jan 25; 290(3):1084–89.

6. Ishida-Takahashi R, Uotani S, Abe T, Degawa-Yamauchi M, Fukushima T, Fujita N, Sakamaki H, Yamasaki H, Yamaguchi Y, Eguchi K. Rapid inhibition of leptin signaling by glucocorticoids in vitro and in vivo. *J Biol Chem.* 2004 May 7; 279(19):19658–64; Leal-Cerro A, Soto A, Martinez MA, Dieguez C, Casanueva FF. Influence of cortisol status on leptin secretion. *Pituitary.* 2001 Jan–Apr; 4(1–2):111–16; Cavagnini F, Croci M, Putignano P, Petroni ML, Invitti C. Glucocorticoids and neuroendocrine function. *Int J Obes Relat Metab Disord.* 2000 Jun; 24 Suppl 2:S77–79.

Chapter 9. Detoxify—and Lose Weight

1. Shore SA, Schwartzman IN, Mellema MS, Flynt L, Imrich A, Johnston RA. Effect of leptin on allergic airway responses in mice. *J Allergy Clin Immunol.* 2005 Jan; 115(1):103–9; Guler N, Kirerleri E, Ones U, Tamay Z, Salmayenli N, Darendeliler F. Leptin: does it have any role in childhood asthma? *J Allergy Clin Immunol.* 2004 Aug; 114(2):254–59.

2. Bornehag CG, Sundell J, Weschler CJ, Sigsgaard T, Lundgren B, Hasselgren M, Hagerhed-Engman L. The association between asthma and allergic symptoms in children and phthalates in house dust: a nested case-control study. *Environ Health Perspect.* 2004 Oct; 112(14):1393–97; Karmaus W, Kuehr J, Kruse H. Infections and atopic disorders in childhood and organochlorine exposure. *Arch Environ Health.*

2001 Nov–Dec; 56(6):485–92; Halken S. Prevention of allergic disease in childhood: clinical and epidemiological aspects of primary and secondary allergy prevention. *Pediatr Allergy Immunol.* 2004 Jun; 15 Suppl 16:4–5, 9–32.

3. Bjorksten B. Environmental factors and respiratory hypersensitivity: experiences from studies in Eastern and Western Europe. *Toxicol Lett.* 1996; 86(2–3):93–98.

4. Tremblay A, Pelletier C, Doucet E, Imbeault P. Thermogenesis and weight loss in obese individuals: a primary association with organochlorine pollution. *Int J Obes Relat Metab Disord.* 2004 Jul; 28(7):936–39; Pelletier C, Doucet E, Imbeault P, Tremblay A. Associations between weight loss–induced changes in plasma organochlorine concentrations, serum T(3) concentration, and resting metabolic rate. *Toxicol Sci.* 2002 May; 67(1):46–51.

5. Moskaug JO, Carlsen H, Myhrstad MC, Blomhoff R. Polyphenols and glutathione synthesis regulation. *Am J Clin Nutr.* 2005 Jan; 81(1 Suppl): 277S–83S; Lampe JW. Spicing up a vegetarian diet: chemopreventive effects of phytochemicals. *Am J Clin Nutr.* 2003 Sep; 78(3 Suppl):579S–83S; Lall SB, Singh B, Gulati K, Seth SD. Role of nutrition in toxic injury. *Indian J Exp Biol.* 1999 Feb; 3 7(2):109–16; Birt DF, Hendrich S, Wang W. Dietary agents in cancer prevention: flavonoids and isoflavonoids. *Pharmacol Ther.* 2001 May–Jun; 90(2–3):157–77; Stahl W, Ale-Agha N, Polidori MC. Nonantioxidant properties of carotenoids. *Biol Chem.* 2002 Mar–Apr; 383(3–4):553–58; Keum YS, Jeong WS, Kong AN. Chemoprevention by isothiocyanates and their underlying molecular signaling mechanisms. *Mutat Res.* 2004 Nov 2; 555(1–2):191–202.

6. Salvi S. Pollution and allergic airways disease. *Curr Opin Allergy Clin Immunol.* 2001 Feb; 1(1):35–41.

7. Oddy WH, de Klerk NH, Kendall GE, Mihrshahi S, Peat JK. Ratio of omega-6 to omega-3 fatty acids and childhood asthma. *J Asthma.* 2004; 41(3):319–26; McKeever TM, Britton J. Diet and asthma. *Am J Respir Crit Care Med.* 2004 Oct 1; 170(7):725–29; Knekt P, Kumpulainen J, Jarvinen R, Rissanen H, Heliovaara M, Reunanen A, Hakulinen T, Aromaa A. Flavonoid intake and risk of chronic diseases. *Am J Clin Nutr.* 2002 Sep; 76(3):560–68; Hartert TV, Peebles RS. Dietary antioxidants and adult asthma. *Curr Opin Allergy Clin Immunol.* 2001 Oct; 1(5):421–29; Shaheen SO, Sterne JA, Thompson RL, Songhurst CE, Margetts BM, Burney PG. Dietary antioxidants and asthma in adults: population-based case-control study. *Am J Respir Crit Care Med.* 2001 Nov 15; 164(10 Pt 1):1823–28; Smit HA, Grievink L, Tabak C. Dietary influences on chronic obstructive lung disease and asthma: a review of the epidemiological evidence. *Proc Nutr Soc.* 1999 May; 58(2):309–19.

8. Inoue H, Kubo M. SOCS proteins in T helper cell differentiation: implications for allergic disorders? *Expert Rev Mol Med.* 2004 Oct 22; 6(22):1–11; Seki Y, Inoue H, Nagata N, Hayashi K, Fukuyama S, Matsumoto K, Komine O, Hamano S, Himeno K, Inagaki-Ohara K, Cacalano N, O'Garra A, Oshida T, Saito H, Johnston JA, Yoshimura A, Kubo M. SOCS-3 regulates onset and maintenance of T(H) 2-mediated allergic responses. *Nat Med.* 2003 Aug; 9(8):1047–54.

ACKNOWLEDGMENTS

We would like to thank our outstanding editor, Susan Berg, whose enthusiastic support made writing this edition such a rewarding experience. We are grateful to the entire team at Rodale for the fantastic job they have done.

We thank the newspaper and magazine editors, television and radio producers, and the reporters and hosts who embraced our healthy message and played such an important role in introducing our book to readers. We would like to thank Rachel Kranz for her important editorial contribution. We have been very fortunate to have our terrific agent, Coleen O'Shea, work with us on this expanded edition.

Christina Galland, beloved wife and mother, brought her extraordinary skills and passion to this book. Jonathan's great-grandmother Helen Savage and grandmother Nellie Oelz cooked from scratch with love and showed us how. Thanks to Jordan Galland for his energy and commitment to helping people achieve better health by teaching them about this diet.

INDEX

Underscored page references indicate boxed text.

About the Author

Leo Galland, M.D., is internationally recognized as a leader in the field of Nutritional Medicine for advancing the scientific understanding of nutritional therapies in the prevention and treatment of chronic disease. A board-certified internist, he is a Fellow of the American College of Physicians and the American College of Nutrition, and is an Honorary Professor of the International College of Nutrition. Dr. Galland is regularly chosen as one of *America's Top Doctors* (Castle Connolly). He is the author of more than thirty scientific articles for publications including the *Journal of the American Medical Association*. He has written textbook chapters for the *Encyclopedia of Human Nutrition, 2nd edition* (Elsevier 2005), *Integrative Medicine, Principles for Practice* (McGraw Hill, 2004), the *Textbook of Natural Medicine, 2nd edition* (McGraw Hill, 2005), and the *Textbook of Functional Medicine* (IFM, 2005). He is also the author of two highly acclaimed books, *Superimmunity for Kids* (Dell, 1989) and *Power Healing* (Random House, 1997).

Dr. Galland received his education at Harvard University and the New York University School of Medicine and trained in internal medicine at the NYU-Bellevue Medical Center. He has held faculty positions at New York University, Rockefeller University, the Albert Einstein College of Medicine, the State University of New York at Stony Brook, and the University of Connecticut. He is the recipient of the Harold W. Harper Award in Preventive Medicine from the American College for Advancement in Medicine and winner of the Linus Pauling Award from the Institute of Functional Medicine and the Clinician Award from the National Nutritional Foods Association (NNFA). Interviews with Dr. Galland and articles about his work have been featured in *Newsweek, Reader's Digest, Redbook, McCall's, Self, Bazaar, Men's Fitness, Allure,* the *New York Times, Daily News,* the *Washington Post,* and many other publications. He has repeatedly appeared as a medical expert on ABC's *Good Morning America,* PBS, Fox News Network, CNN, and MSNBC, as well as the Christian and Trinity Broadcasting Networks and dozens of local affiliates of the major broadcast networks. He is currently the Director of the Foundation for Integrated Medicine (www.mdheal.org) and maintains a private practice in New York.

Jonathan Galland is a health writer and columnist for newspapers, magazines, and major Web sites. He is frequently interviewed as a weight loss and health expert on the radio and has appeared on *Martha Stewart Living Radio*. His work has been featured on the covers of *Fitness, Glamour,* and *Women's World* and in publications such as the *Washington Post, Body and Soul, Self,* and the *Wall Street Journal.* Jonathan's newsletter at www.fatresistancediet.com encourages and inspires readers from around the world. He has collaborated with international editors to introduce *The Fat Resistance Diet* to Italy and Japan where it has been translated and published in Milan as *La Dieta Galland* and in Tokyo as *Dr. Galland's Metabolic Diet.* Jonathan is also active in community outreach, providing his health articles to diverse community organizations through the Foundation for Integrated Medicine at www.mdheal.org.

Join the Resistance!

Stay Connected for Success with the Fat Resistance Diet

Are you ready to supercharge your metabolism, lose weight, and optimize your well-being? Thousands of readers from around the world have "joined the resistance" at our Web site, www.fatresistancediet.com. Simply go to the Web site and sign up for our newsletter. Readers tell us our newsletters are a wonderful way to stay connected and on track with our diet. The reader testimonials in this book are from our newsletter subscribers, demonstrating what a powerful tool this is.

Receive the latest news and health information, such as:

- Special announcements of upcoming radio and TV appearances by the authors
- Seasonal fruit and vegetable buying guide
- How to enjoy Fat Resistance Foods and recipes
- Resources and links
- Updates on Fat Resistance in the news

We need your help to introduce the important health benefits of the Fat Resistance Diet to the people who need it. You can make a difference in your community and help others lose weight and get healthy. Together we can fight the obesity crisis and make the world a healthier place.

- Tell your family, friends and co-workers about our diet. Share with them the exciting ideas from the book, the recipes, and Jonathan's Kitchen Tips.
- Forward our newsletter to everyone on your e-mail list.
- Request that your local library obtain a copy of *The Fat Resistance Diet*. Requests are an important way libraries choose books.
- Let your local newspaper, radio station, or TV station know about our book. They are always looking for new stories and have shown great interest in *The Fat Resistance Diet*. Have them contact us at PR@fatresistancediet.com.